OphthoBook
QUESTIONS
VOLUME ONE

ALSO BY TIMOTHY ROOT

OphthoBook - A Student's Guide to the Eye
www.OphthoBook.com

Root Eye Dictionary - A Guide to Common Eye Problems
www.RootEyeDictionary.com

My First Cataract - A Patient's Guide to Cataract Surgery
www.MyFirstCataract.com

Benjamin Impossible - Diabolical Genius with Kung Fu Grip
www.BenjaminImpossible.com

OphthoBook
QUESTIONS
VOLUME ONE

Timothy Root, M.D.

Copyright © 2016 by Timothy D. Root
All rights reserved. This book or any portion thereof
may not be reproduced or used in any manner whatsoever
without the express written permission of the publisher
except for the use of brief quotations in a book review.

Printed in the United States of America

First Printing, 2016

www.OphthoBook.com

CHAPTERS

Introduction	1
Chapter 1: Anatomy	5
Chapter 2: Cataract & Lens	25
Chapter 3: Cornea	53
Chapter 4: General	69
Chapter 5: Glaucoma	83
Chapter 6: Infection	101
Chapter 7: Lids & Lacrimation	117
Chapter 8: Neuro	133
Chapter 9: Optics	155
Chapter 10: Pediatrics	167
Chapter 11: Retina	183
Chapter 12: Trauma	203
Chapter 13: Uveitis	219
Conclusion	229

INTRODUCTION

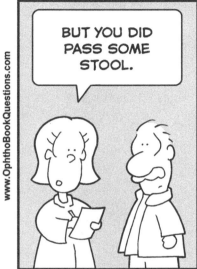
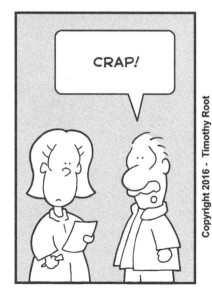
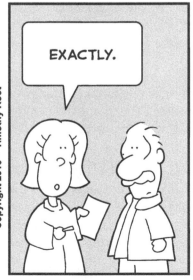

INTRODUCTION

Welcome fellow student ... or perhaps I should say *pupil*! You've just picked up the greatest question book ever written for the beginning eye student. This book contains over 300 multiple choice questions, sampling every subspecialty within our field. It's perfect for the struggling student or technician trying to get ahead!

Are you a crazy person who likes *hard* books?
Before you continue, ask yourself a couple of questions:

1. Do you revel in esoteric exam questions and spend your nights playing trivia in bars?

2. Are you a student "gunner" hated by your classmates and looking to one-up your peers with your mastery of minutia?

3. Do minor typos and grammatical errors drive you insane and compel you to write scathing book reviews?

If you answered "yes" to any of these questions, this is the *wrong* book for you. You see, this is a SIMPLE book, designed for the NEW student. These questions are intended for "normal people" trying to get a grip on the fundamentals of ophthalmology. This is NOT an advanced book designed to master fine details.

This book is appropriate for medical students, optometry students, and eye technicians scrambling to learn the basics as quickly as possible. The material within these pages is BASIC! Experienced residents and practicing doctors will find this series too easy.

Why bother with a basic question book?
As a medical student, I found ophthalmology intimidating and difficult to grasp. Rather than teach me basics, my preceptors seemed to imply that EVERYTHING was important. This was obviously not true. I remember being sent to the library to spend hours studying the effects of homocysteinemia on the eye - a condition that I haven't seen ONCE during my residency training, or

in my busy private practice. An unfocussed, tangential approach like this is paralyzing and inefficient for the new student.

Professional students (that's YOU) know that old exams and test questions are invaluable for honing in on the "important" material (and for scoring well on exams). Unfortunately, as a student I simply couldn't *find* any eye question books appropriate for my level of training. The internet was barely just starting, and the classic ophthalmology question books (Chern, Mass Eye & Ear, ProVision) were written at an advanced level to help experienced eye doctors pass their board certification exams. These massive tomes were filled with obscure facts bearing little relevance to real life and just weren't appropriate for the beginning student.

Hopefully, this book will be more useful and appropriate for YOUR level.

The unconventional layout?
Question books normally force you to flip pages to read the answer key in the back of the book. This keeps you from "cheating" as you take the virtual test. This sounds great in theory, but it quickly becomes tedious. The fastest way to learn a skill is through IMMEDIATE feedback. That's why I've placed each answer immediately AFTER each question. I've also included a great deal of detail with each answer so that you don't have to reference outside books. And I've added some humor, silly answers and cartoons, all in an attempt to add a little spice and make the book easier to swallow.

Enjoy it and send me money!
I encourage you to purchase the printed version of this book to support this project. The receipts allow me to donate books to students and to keep the website running. If you ARE reading the printed (paid) version of this book - I salute you!

Thanks a bunch!
Tim Root

CHAPTER 1
ANATOMY

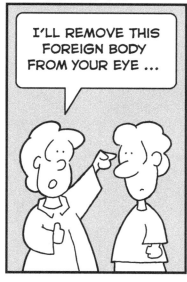
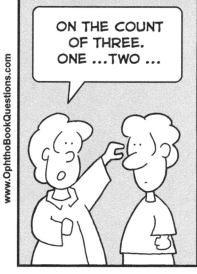
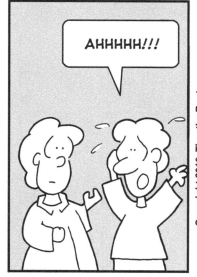
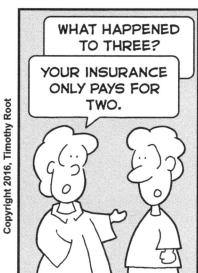

ANATOMY
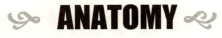
25 Questions

1. The eye socket is also known as the:
A. pestle
B. cradle
C. orbit
D. eyehole

The eye socket is called the orbit, so the correct answer is (c). The "orbit" is a common term. For example, when people have an infection behind the eye, this is commonly called an "orbital cellulitis." A break of one of the bones surrounding the eyeball is also called an "orbital fracture." A mortar and pestle are a small bowl and grinding wand used to pulverize medicines and herbs - these days, they're mostly used in Mexican restaurants to make guacamole! Cradles are used with babies. "Eyehole" is wrong, but also funny.

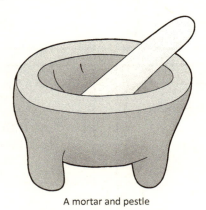

A mortar and pestle

2. The limbus is the intersection of the:
A. iris and trabecular meshwork
B. cornea and trabecular meshwork
C. sclera and cornea
D. conjunctiva and sclera

The correct answer is (c). The limbus is the intersection of the cornea and the sclera. Externally, it is the ring where the "white" of the eye touches the "colored portion" of the eye. Limbus is a common anatomic landmark used for describing the location of other lesions. For example, you might say that a patient has a corneal ulcer near the limbus at 6 o'clock. There are also limbal stem cells that are important for the regrowth of surface epithelium following a corneal abrasion.

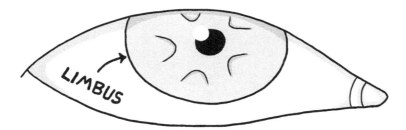

The terms "limbus" and "limbal" are commonly used in ophthalmology to help describe the location of lesions, such as limbal ulcers and abrasions.

3. How many extraocular eye muscles attach to the sclera?
A. 3
B. 4
C. 5
D. 6

There are six extraocular muscles that control eye movement and each of them connects to the sclera. The correct answer is therefore (d). The four rectus muscles each attach to the sclera at a point 5-8 mm back from the limbus. These insertion distances form the famous "Spiral of Tillaux." This fact becomes important during muscle surgery, but don't kill yourself memorizing the numbers at this point. The superior oblique muscle travels through a trochlear pulley, near the nose, before inserting on the back of the sclera. The inferior oblique also inserts on the posterior sclera at the back of the eye near the macula.

CHAPTER 1: ANATOMY

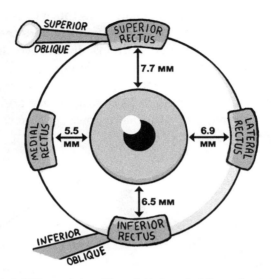

Spiral of Tillaux ... not terribly useful to know in daily practice, but a classic test question on ophthalmology board tests.

4. The extraocular muscles all attach to the orbital apex, <u>except</u> for the:
A. superior rectus
B. superior oblique
C. inferior rectus
D. inferior oblique

The correct answer is (d). All of the extraocular muscles, even the long and circuitous superior oblique, originate at the back of the eye socket (the apex) at a circular ring of tissue called the annulus of Zinn. The only muscle that doesn't fit this pattern is the inferior oblique muscle, which actually originates from the floor of the orbit.

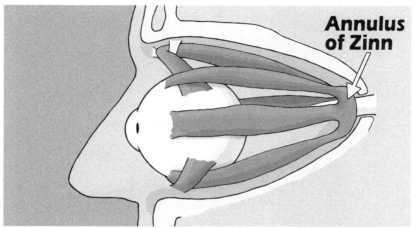

Almost all the eye muscles attach at the annulus of Zinn. This includes the superior oblique. The inferior oblique is the weird one, as it originates on the orbital floor. Fortunately, this odd muscle has the least clinical relevance.

5. What is the purpose of the meibomian glands?
A. oil production
B. antimicrobial production
C. accessory tear production
D. lutein conversion

The correct answer is (a). The primary purpose of the meibomian glands is to produce oil that is slowly released into the tear film. This oil forms the superficial lipid layer of the tear film, and it is important for maintaining surface tension and decreasing the effects of evaporation. The meibomian orifices can be seen running along the inner edge of the eyelid under low-power microscope. The oil they produce can be squeezed out with a Q-tip. Other glands, such as the accessory tear glands within the conjunctiva, produce the aqueous component of our tears that includes natural antimicrobials. Lutein is a plant pigment found in high concentration within the retina. It is often used as a supplement in eye vitamins.

CHAPTER 1: ANATOMY

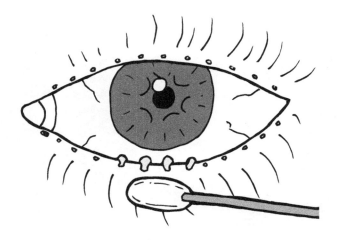

Meibomian gland being expressed with Q-tip. Normally, this oil comes out clear like vegetable oil. However, in people with blepharitis, the oil oozes out slowly like toothpaste.

6. Which layer is deepest?
A. conjunctiva
B. Tenon's fascia
C. episclera
D. sclera

The correct answer here is (d). The sclera is the deepest layer. The sclera is the collagen tissue that forms the white wall of the eye. The episclera is a thin layer of tissue and blood vessels immediately overlying the sclera. You can see episcleral blood vessels during an eye exam: they are the deep, non-moving blood vessels on the surface of the white eyeball. Tenon's fascia is a diffuse white tissue that exists outside of the eyeball but still under the surface of the conjunctival tissue. You can't really *see* Tenon's during an eye exam, but it is quite obvious during any eye surgery that involves cutting through the conjunctiva. When we cut through the conjunctiva (to get to the eyeball or muscles underneath) Tenon's looks and acts like wet tissue paper. It swells up with water when we make injections under the conjunctiva, and it tends to get in the way. We often have to scrape Tenon's away with a flat blade to achieve clean access to the sclera underneath.

7. Behind the iris sits the:
A. scleral ring
B. ciliary body
C. ciliary ganglion
D. scleral spur

The correct answer is (b). Just behind the iris sits a band of muscle called the ciliary body. The ciliary body is a sphincter-like muscle, embryologically related to the iris. This ciliary body muscle focuses the lens and it also produces aqueous fluid. In contrast, the ciliary ganglion is a nexus of nerves behind the eye that is part of the parasympathetic system controlling pupil constriction. Damage to this ganglion causes Adie's syndrome (pupil dilation secondary to loss of parasympathetic input). The scleral "spur" is a protrusion of the sclera into the anterior chamber in front of the iris. This spur serves as insertion point for internal eye muscles (ciliary body/iris), and is only seen during gonioscopy of the angle. A scleral "ring" is a ring of bone found in many birds, reptiles, and dinosaur fossils ... its purpose is to strengthen and protect the eye. It is not found in humans as we have no bones in our eye.

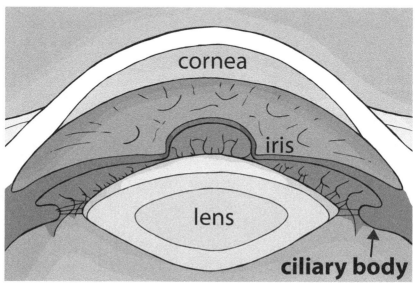

The ciliary body sits underneath/behind the iris. It can't be seen during a normal eye exam unless the patient dilates REALLY wide or if you use a gonio lens to look behind the iris.

CHAPTER 1: ANATOMY

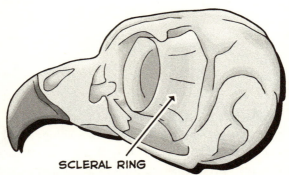

This is the scleral ring bone in an owl skull. Owls are unique as their eyes completely fill their eye sockets and don't move. They have to move their entire head to look around. Watch my comparative anatomy lecture if you find this kind of thing interesting!

8. How long is the eye?
A. 18 mm
B. 24 mm
C. 33 mm
D. size isn't everything

The correct answer is (b). The eye is about 24 mm long. If you have a tough time remembering this, just think of the eye as being about 1 inch (2.54 cm long) and you'll be close. There is, of course, some variation in eye size. On average, myopic (nearsighted) people have longer eyes, and hyperopic (farsighted) have shorter eyes. There are also conditions such as nanophthalmos, where people have a very short eye (20 mm). Other conditions, such as microphthalmos, arise from embryologic malformations - these conditions are rare, and are more than you need to know at this point. The main reason that we care about ocular length is during the calculation of implant power prior to cataract surgery. A short eye needs a stronger implant power in order to focus objects on the retina.

9. What is the volume of the eye?
A. 1 cc
B. 6 cc
C. 15 cc
D. 60 cc

The correct answer is (b). The volume of the entire eye is close to six cubic centimeters. It can be calculated using basic geometry if you know the length of the eye. Of this volume, the vitreous gel in the back makes up about 4cc. The anterior chamber takes up only 0.3 cc. These numbers aren't super high-yield at the moment, but I want to emphasize how small the eye is. When retina doctors inject medications inside the vitreous, they do so using those tiny 1cc TB-syringes and they can only inject 0.1 to 0.2 cc at a time. Even then, the pressure can rise quickly because the eye doesn't expand, and may require a paracentesis of extra aqueous from the anterior chamber to keep the eye pressure normal. The orbit itself (eye socket) has a volume of only 30 cc - about the same as a ping-pong ball. This extra space is filled with eye muscles and supporting fat-pads that cushion the eye.

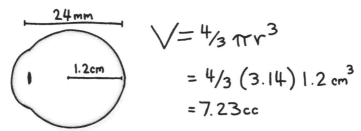

You remember the calculation for the volume of a sphere, don't you?

10. The purpose of the ciliary body is to:
A. focus the eye
B. produce fluid
C. both of the above
D. neither of the above

The correct answer is (c). The ciliary body sits behind the iris. It holds the lens in place by suspending the lens with zonules. The ciliary body contracts like a sphincter muscle, relaxing the zonular tension, allowing the lens to become rounder. This process is called accommodation, and is necessary to see up-close. The ciliary body also produces the aqueous fluid that fills and nourishes the front part of the eye.

CHAPTER 1: ANATOMY

11. The blind spot occurs because of the location of the:
A. optic nerve
B. macula
C. foveola
D. fovea

The correct answer here is (a). The blind spot corresponds to the location of the optic nerve. The optic nerve insertion is the only point in the retina not covered by photoreceptors. The macula is the pigmented area in our vision responsible for central vision. The fovea is located in the middle of the macula. This is where our finest central vision occurs. The foveola is an anatomic term that is rarely used in clinical practice. It is the "pit" in the middle of the fovea that can be seen on cross-section scans of the retinal surface (such as with an OCT scan).

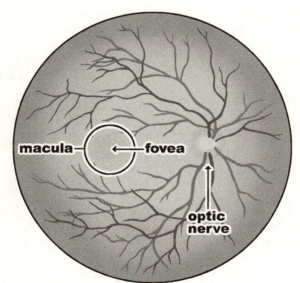

The basic retina landmarks

12. How many chambers are there in the eye?
A. 2
B. 3
C. 4
D. 5

The correct answer is (b). There are actually three chambers in the eye. The anterior chamber, in the front, is filled with aqueous fluid. The vitreous chamber, in the back, is filled with vitreous gel. There is a third chamber, the "posterior" chamber, which is located in between. This posterior chamber is located immediately behind the iris but still in front of the lens, and is filled with aqueous fluid produced by the ciliary body. This small chamber is important in the discussion of cataract surgery. We call our lens implants PCIOL (posterior chamber intraocular lenses) in order to differentiate them from older ACIOL (anterior chamber intraocular lenses). Also, when people have acute glaucoma, we use a laser to punch a hole through the iris to equalize the pressure between the anterior and posterior chambers. This allows the iris diaphragm to rotate back into a normal position, opening up the drainage angle.

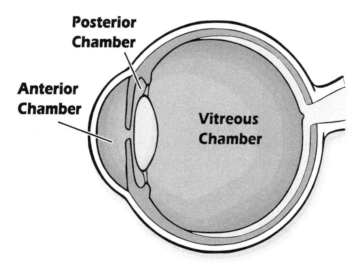

There are actually three chambers in the eye!

13. Avascular structures in the eye include all, <u>except</u>:
A. cornea
B. lens
C. vitreous
D. conjunctiva

CHAPTER 1: ANATOMY

The answer here is (d). The conjunctiva is a vascular structure ... you can see the blood vessels running through it when looking in the mirror. The cornea and lens are living tissues but have no blood vessels, as this would interfere with the transmission of light. Instead, these structures receive their nutrition from aqueous inside the eye. The cornea also receives nutrition and oxygen from the tear film. The vitreous is a cavity filled with a gelatinous fluid ... this is not a metabolically active structure, so it doesn't require a vasculature. However, abnormal blood vessels CAN grow into the vitreous gel with conditions like ROP (retinopathy of prematurity) or proliferative diabetic retinopathy. These abnormal vessels can bleed and scar, resulting in vitreous hemorrhage and retinal detachment.

14. What type of collagen is the sclera made of?
A. type 1
B. type 2
C. type 3
D. type 4

The correct answer is (b). The majority of the cornea and the sclera that make up the outer eyeball are made of type 2 collagen. This "fact" borders on unimportant, but recognize that it could show up on a test. The other collagen type that you should be aware of is type 4 collagen, which is the collagen found in basement membranes. The outer lens capsule is made of basement membrane, as is Descemet's membrane (which is the basement membrane for the corneal endothelium). Relevance? Not much in daily practice, unless you are a pathologist.

15. The retina terminates at the:
A. lamina papyracea
B. ora serrata
C. retinaculum ora
D. equator

The correct answer is (b). The retina covers the inside of the eye like film in a camera or wallpaper on a wall. The edge of the retina is called the ora serrata because it has a serrated, or scalloped, appearance. It is difficult to view the retina in the far periphery. Often, inspection requires scleral depression (indenting the eye) or a 3-mirror gonio lens. The lamina papyracea is a "paper thin" wall that forms the medial wall of the orbit. It is formed by the ethmoid bone and is susceptible to breaking with blunt ocular trauma. The "retinaculum ora" is a made-up phrase, though you can find "retinaculum" throughout the body, as this is a sheath of tissue that serves to help stabilize tendons.

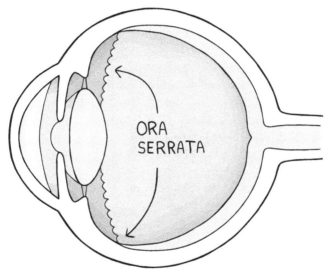

The ora can be difficult to visualize, even with the indirect scope. Sometimes you have to actually indent the eye with a Q-tip (scleral depression) to push it into view

16. The lens is suspended by:
A. trochlea
B. zonules
C. Whitnall's ligament
D. tarsal plate

The correct answer is (b). The lens is suspended by zonules attached to the periphery like trampoline springs. These zonules can break after trauma or during cataract surgery. This is called a zonular dehiscence and can create lens dislocation. The trochlea is a fibrous pulley near the nose that changes the direction of force exerted by the superior oblique muscle. Whitnall's ligament (not high yield at this point in your studies) is located above the eye, and helps the levator muscle raise the upper eyelid. The tarsal plate is located in the eyelid.

17. Retinal ganglion nerves pass through what structure before forming the optic nerve?
A. lamina papyracea
B. cribriform plate
C. lamina cribrosa
D. lamina corian

The answer is (c). The ganglion nerve cells that run along the surface of the retina dive down at the optic disc, through the lamina cribrosa, to form the optic nerve. The lamina cribrosa looks like a round plate with tiny holes through which the nerves pass through as they exit the globe. These little holes can sometimes be seen during a dilated exam, especially in people with glaucomatous nerve loss. The lamina papyracea is the "paper thin" wall of the ethmoid bone. The cribriform plate is the spot where olfactory nerves pass through the skull to enter the nose. "Lamina corian" is something that I made up: Corian is a man-made plastic material created by DuPont and is used to make countertops. My kitchen has Corian countertops, and my wife wants us to upgrade to heat-resistant granite.

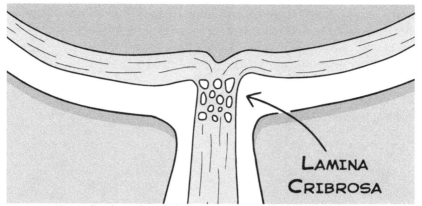
Nerves dive down through the lamina cribrosa to form the optic nerve.

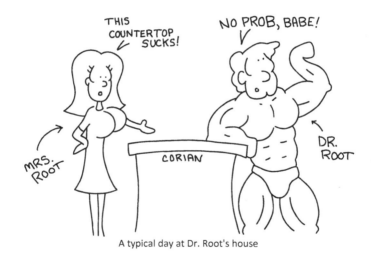
A typical day at Dr. Root's house

18. The medial wall of the orbit is formed by the:
A. maxillary bone
B. zygomatic bone
C. frontal bone
D. ethmoid bone

The correct answer is (d). The ethmoid sinuses make up the medial wall of the eye socket. This ethmoid bone is quite thin and is called the lamina papyracea (paper wall). Despite its thinness, the medial wall rarely breaks during trauma thanks to extensive sinus buttressing. However, ethmoid sinus infections CAN erode through this wall, causing a potentially deadly orbital cellulitis. The bones that make up the other "walls" of the orbit can be easily deduced from the surrounding anatomy. The roof is formed by the frontal bone, the lateral wall by the zygomatic bone, and the floor of the orbit is formed by the maxillary bone.

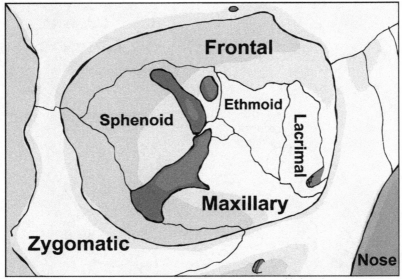

The bones look scary to memorize, right? The only bones that are likely to be important to an eye doctor are the maxillary and ethmoid bones. Don't even worry about the sphenoid wings and palatine bone (not labeled) unless you have OCD.

19. Tears drain into the nose via all, <u>except</u>:
A. punctum
B. nasolacrimal sac
C. canaliculi
D. lacrimal gland

The correct answer is (d). The tears drain into the nose via the nasolacrimal system. This is the pathway from the puncta, through the canaliculi, the nasolacrimal sac, and finally the nasolacrimal duct into the nose. The lacrimal gland is located in the upper eyelid/orbit and is responsible for the production of reflexive tearing.

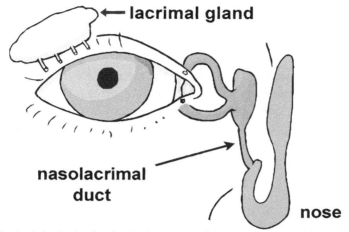

The lacrimal gland is that big gland in the upper eyelid. You can't see it well during an eye exam, and it is rarely clinically relevant as it only produces reflex tears.

20. What is the layer of skin on the inside of the eyelids called?
A. eyelid mucosa
B. bulbar conjunctiva
C. palpebral conjunctiva
D. lacrimal conjunctiva

The correct answer is (c). The conjunctiva is the tissue that forms the surface of the eyeball. The portion on the eyeball itself is referred to as the bulbar conjunctiva. This conjunctiva loops forward and forms the inner surface of the eyelids, where it is called the palpebral conjunctiva. This is relevant, as the palpebral conjunctiva can become irritated from infection or contact lens overwear, leading to the formation of small bumps (papillae or follicles) on the inner lids. There is no such thing as the lacrimal conjunctiva. "Eyelid mucosa" is not a term I've ever heard, even though it kind of makes sense.

CHAPTER 1: ANATOMY

21. What muscle "opens" the upper eyelid?
A. orbicularis oculi
B. orbicularis domini
C. orbicularis palpebrae
D. levator palpebrae

The correct answer is (d). The levator palpebrae is the muscle that raises the upper eyelid by pulling upward on the tarsal plate. Like most of the extraocular muscles, the levator muscle is controlled by the third cranial nerve. Most cases of ptosis (droopy eyelid) are repaired by shortening the levator. The orbicularis oculi is the ring of muscles that close the eye. There is no such thing as the orbicularis domini or orbicularis palpebrae.

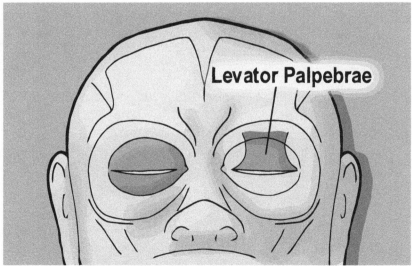

The levator muscle pulls the eyelid open. The orbicularis closes the eye.

22. The vitreous is primarily responsible for:
A. retinal nutrition
B. refraction
C. generation of eye pressure
D. none of the above

The correct answer is (d). The vitreous is the gel that fills most of the eye. Its purpose is to maintain the shape of the eye and to remain clear so that light can pass through it unimpeded. The vitreous has no role in retinal nutrition, refraction, or eye pressure. The eye's pressure is mainly a function of the production and drainage of aqueous fluid in the front part of the eye.

23. All of the following can be examined with the slit-lamp microscope, except:
A. cornea
B. trabecular meshwork
C. retina
D. axilla

The correct answer is (d). The slit-lamp microscope is primarily used to examine the front part of the eye, though the retina can be viewed with accessory lenses. A mirrored gonio lens allows the trabecular meshwork to be visualized as well. The slit-lamp is not great for examining the axilla (arm pit).

24. The iris contains how many muscles?
A. 1
B. 2
C. 3
D. 4

The answer is (b). The iris is composed of two muscles ... the iris dilator and the iris constrictor muscles. The constrictor muscle is a sphincter-like muscle, located around the pupil. It is controlled by the parasympathetic system and constricts with bright light and when focusing on near objects. The dilator muscle is located radially and controlled by the sympathetic system to "pull" the pupil open. When we dilate patients in our office, we usually use two types of drops: one, phenylephrine, is a direct sympathomimetic that stimulates the radial retractor muscles to dilate the pupil.

CHAPTER 1: ANATOMY

Tropicamide is the other - it is a parasympathetic blocker that allows the iris sphincter to relax.

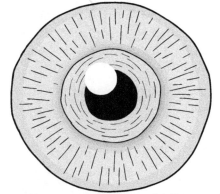

Inner sphincter muscle and outer radial dilator muscle

25. How many layers are there in the lens?
A. one
B. two
C. three
D. four

Three layers comprise the lens. These consist of the outer capsule, the middle cortex, and the central nucleus. When we perform cataract surgery, we vacuum out the inner two layers and leave the capsule behind to hold the new plastic implant. The correct answer is therefore (c).

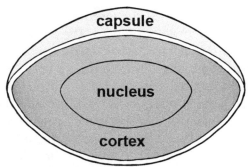

The lens has three layers ... like a peanut M&M candy

CHAPTER 2
CATARACT & LENS

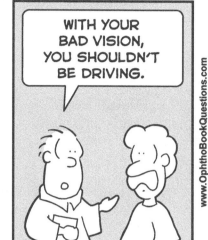
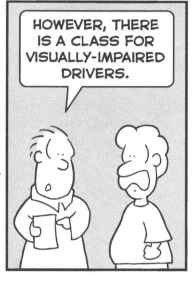
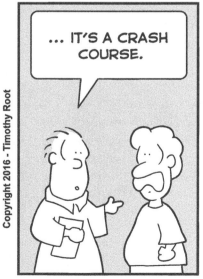

CATARACT & LENS

34 Questions

1. A person undergoes cataract surgery and has an implant placed in each eye. This person is now considered:
A. phakic
B. neuphakic
C. pseudophakic
D. aphakic

The correct answer is (c). A person with a prosthetic implant in their eye is considered pseudophakic. If you have your natural lens, you are considered to be phakic, and if you have no lens/implant you are aphakic. Most people who are aphakic have a history of trauma to their eye, or had their cataract surgery 40+ years ago before the advent of good intraocular lenses. "Aphakes" require thick "aphakic spectacles" or contact lenses in order to see well. Neuphakic is not a real term.

2. Modern cataract surgery is usually performed:
A. extracapsular
B. intracapsular
C. intercapsular
D. innerspace

The correct answer is (a). Modern cataract surgery is performed as extracapsular surgery, which means that the lens capsule is left behind as a support structure to facilitate the placement of a new implant. Intracapsular surgery is an older technique in which the cataract and capsule were removed in one piece. With this older method, a cryoprobe was stuck to the lens and the entire cataract was pulled out, ripping the zonular support springs entirely. The problem with intracapsular surgery is that this leaves no place to secure a new implant, except in the anterior chamber (on top of the iris). There is no such thing as <u>inter</u>capsular surgery. InnerSpace is a 1987 movie staring Martin Short and Dennis Quaid, where Quaid finds himself shrunk inside a tiny spaceship and injected into Short's bloodstream.

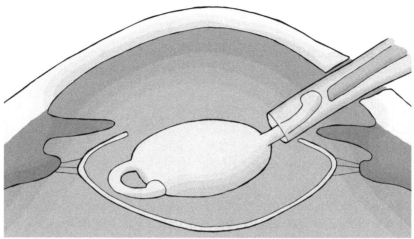

With extracapsular surgery, the lens capsule is left in place to support the placement of an implanted plastic lens.

3. Extracapsular cataract extraction can be performed using all of the following techniques, except:
A. with phacoemulsification
B. without phacoemulsification
C. using a cryoprobe
D. tunneling through the sclera

The correct answer is (c). If you read the last question, this should be pretty obvious. Extracapsular cataract surgery involves leaving the outer capsule of a cataract in place while removing the inner cortex and nucleus. The removal of the internal cataract can be performed in several ways. Modern surgery involves using a phacoemulsification tip that vibrates at ultrasonic frequencies, breaking up the nucleus and allowing it to be vacuumed out. If a person has a very dense cataract, however, these ultrasonic vibrations may not be capable of pulverizing the nucleus. In these cases, the nucleus is removed from the eye in one giant piece through a larger incision. Most modern surgeons make their incisions through the clear cornea. When a larger incision is required, it's often better to tunnel through the sclera near the limbus as this creates less corneal distortion afterwards. The cryoprobe is only used with older intracapsular surgery.

4. An eye doctor tells you they had to perform a cataract surgery "as an extracap." This implies the surgery was performed:
A. using phacoemulsification
B. through a large incision
C. through a small incision
D. they had to "pop a cap" twice

The correct answer is (b). Technically, all modern cataract surgery is performed as an extracapsular extraction, as the capsule is always left behind. However, with the advent of modern phacoemulsification, the term "extracap" is usually used now to describe the removal of the nucleus in one piece through a larger incision. This is required when the nucleus is too dense to safely remove with ultrasound, or if there are complications in which the capsule's integrity is questionable and we're afraid we're going to "drop a lens" into the vitreous cavity. In these cases, a larger incision is created, and a small lens loop (essentially a spoon) is slid under the nucleus. The nucleus is then gently pulled out of the eye. Hopefully, the capsular "bag" remains intact so that an implant can be placed back into the capsule. If not, the implant can be placed on top of the capsule (under the iris) or an anterior chamber lens may be placed on top of the iris. Extracapsular surgery is rare in the U.S. (about one for every two thousand cases in my own private practice). It is more common with complicated cases (residency training hospitals) and extremely common in developing countries.

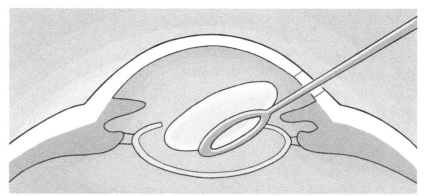

"Extracapsular surgery" usually implies nucleus removal without phacoemulsification. It is performed through a larger incision.

5. Cataract removal is recommended when:
A. vision has dropped to 20/50
B. the cataract looks "ripe"
C. no longer legal to drive
D. ADLs become affected

The correct answer is (d). Cataract surgery has become refined and safe enough that it is commonly performed when ADLs (activities of daily living) are being negatively affected by poor vision. This measurement is relative, however. I've had pilots with 20/25 vision who needed their cataracts out as they couldn't perform their job secondary to nighttime glare. I've also had patients with 20/200 vision that we leave alone because they aren't driving and are content with their visual acuity. The concept of a cataract being "ripe" probably stemmed from the older days of surgery, when the procedure was much riskier and the cataract was removed in one piece. In this scenario, eye doctors would prefer the cataract to be dense so that it could be removed in one piece without falling apart. Now that we remove cataracts by breaking them up, it is better to remove them BEFORE they become too hard and "ripe."

CHAPTER 2: CATARACT & LENS

6. Methods to grade the severity of Fuchs' dystrophy prior to cataract surgery include all, <u>except</u>:
A. specular count
B. pachymetry
C. morning acuity
D. guttaemetry

The correct answer is (d). Fuchs' dystrophy is a common condition in which patients have less corneal endothelial cells than normal. The endothelial cells are very important as they act as "pumps" to keep the cornea dry and clear. These cells don't replicate when damaged. Fortunately, most of us are born with so many of these cells that it's not a problem. People with Fuchs' may have problems after cataract surgery, however, as a certain percentage of endothelial cells are damaged with any intraocular surgery. This can lead to corneal cloudiness after surgery, necessitating corneal transplant in order to replace this damaged endothelial layer. During pre-operative consultation, we attempt to estimate the possibility of Fuchs' complications. Specular microscopy is a method for actually visualizing the endothelial cells under a microscope and counting the number of cells (cell count) and their morphology. It is rarely performed these days (I've never done it, myself) but may still be performed by some cornea doctors at teaching institutions. Pachymetry (measurement of the corneal thickness) is an easy test to measure how thick (wet) the cornea is prior to surgery. A thick cornea pre-operatively is an ominous sign. Fuchs' dystrophy tends to cause blurriness in the morning, as evaporation helps dry the cornea later in the day. If your patient ALREADY has blurriness in the morning secondary to Fuchs', it will almost assuredly be worse after surgery. Guttae (often called guttata) are divots on the back of the cornea seen during routine eye exam and are prevalent with Fuchs'. There isn't really a standard way of measuring these bumps, so "guttaemetry" is a made-up term.

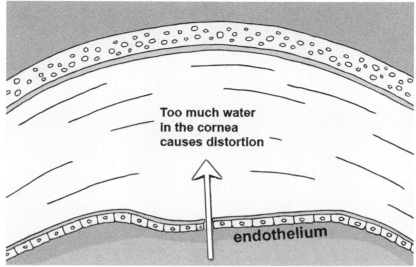

With Fuchs' dystrophy, the endothelium is not able to remove fluid from the cornea fast enough and the cornea stroma becomes cloudy.

7. Pseudoexfoliation syndrome increases the risk of <u>what</u> during surgery?
A. dropped lens
B. glaucoma
C. corneal edema
D. chamber shallowing

The correct answer is (a). Pseudoexfoliation syndrome (also called PXF or PEX) is a condition where a white, flaky material forms on the surface of the lens/cataract. This material has a composition similar to that of basement membrane tissue. It can be seen as a flaky crust on the front surface of the lens during the slit-lamp exam. As the iris dilates and constricts over a life time, this pseudoexfoliation material can rub off and become trapped in the trabecular meshwork. This increases the risk of glaucoma. Pseudoexfoliation material can also attach to and weaken the zonular springs that support the lens. During cataract surgery, these zonules can break and cause the cataract to dislocate and drop into the vitreous cavity. PXF is a common finding in Scandinavian countries like Norway and Sweden. The other answers are wrong: PXF doesn't cause glaucoma *during* surgery, nor does it cause corneal edema.

Chamber shallowing is associated more often with "acute" angle-closure glaucoma, which doesn't occur during surgery either.

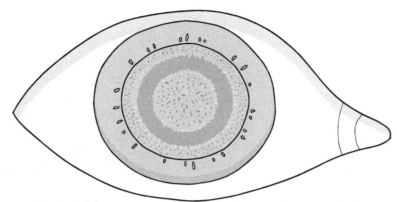

Rings of pseudoexfoliation material can be seen on the lens surface. Watch for glaucoma and be careful during cataract surgery! Those zonules might be weak!

8. Which of the following is <u>least</u> troublesome during cataract surgery?
A. poor pupil dilation
B. brunescent cataract
C. pseudoexfoliation
D. pigment dispersion syndrome

The correct answer is (d). Pigment dispersion syndrome (PDS) occurs mostly in young, near-sighted people, when the iris bows backwards and rubs on the lens and zonules. This releases pigment into the anterior chamber, clogging the trabecular meshwork and potentially leading to glaucoma. This condition often "burns out" as we get older and it is not associated with cataracts or problems during surgery. On the other hand, poor pupil dilation and dense, brunescent (brown) cataracts are the major cause of surgical complications. Pseudoexfoliation syndrome is a condition in which a flaky material forms on the lens and zonules. This material can rub off and cause glaucoma, but it also weakens the zonules and can lead to breakage (zonular dehiscence) and lens dislocation during and after surgery.

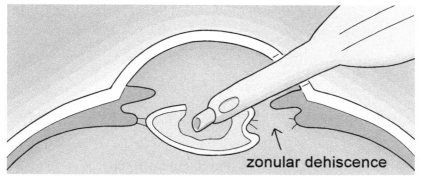

A zonular dehiscence can occur with dense cataracts because of the increased manipulation needed to break up the nucleus. Pseudoexfoliation syndrome can also weaken the zonules and cause them to break.

9. A PSC is:
A. type of cataract
B. an after-cataract
C. type of surgery center
D. embryologic suture line

The correct answer is (a). PSC stands for posterior subcapsular cataract. This is a cataract opacity that occurs at the back of the lens and looks like white sand or bread crumbs plastered against the back, inner surface of the lens capsule. This type of cataract forms rapidly and is most common among younger patients, steroid users, and diabetics. The posterior location of PSC cataracts causes more visual complaints than anterior opacities, possibly because the overall "nodal point" of the eye's lens system is located at the back of the lens (thus, more light rays are affected). PSC cataracts are generally easy to remove, as these patients are young and the nucleus is soft. The other answers here are incorrect. ASC is an abbreviation for "ambulatory surgery center" (or possibly a rare anterior subcapsular cataract). The lens does have embryologic suture lines; these may be seen with careful examination using the slit-lamp microscope. This finding is inconsequential, however, and rarely mentioned. An "after cataract" is called a PCO (posterior capsular opacity) or less commonly OPC (opacification of the posterior capsule). Memorizing the difference between a PSC and PCO used to drive me crazy as student, so here's a drawing:

CHAPTER 2: CATARACT & LENS

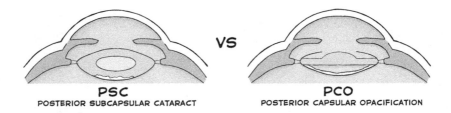

10. Lens implants are calculated by measuring:
A. keratometry and axial length
B. pachymetry and horizontal depth
C. axial length and anterior lens depth
D. corneal power and current refraction

The correct answer is (a). There have been many attempts to calculate the correct implant power needed with lens replacement surgery. The most consistent measurements used are the axial length (the length of the eye from cornea to retina) and keratometry (the steepness of the cornea). Here is the "SRK equation" commonly used prior to surgery. Don't try memorizing this ... it's not high yield (yet).

Implant Power = A-constant - 0.9 (average Kornea steepness) - 2.5 (Axial length)

There are many different implant styles, manufacturers, and types of plastic available. To work in the above equation, each implant comes with a pre-calculated "A constant." Don't kill yourself with formulas ... just realize that prior to surgery, we need to get our patients "A's and K's" (Axial length and Keratometry of cornea).

11. "Potential vision" in a patient with dense cataracts can be estimated with all of the following techniques, except:
A. color detection
B. pinhole PAM
C. light projection
D. contrast sensitivity

The best answer here is (d). During a pre-operative evaluation we attempt to estimate how much vision a patient may regain after surgery. This is especially important in people with coexisting retina damage or in individuals whose retina cannot be visualized (such as with dense, white cataracts). The most common method for estimating retinal vision is with a PAM (potential acuity meter). This gadget attaches to the slit-lamp and shoots beams of light (or an eye chart) through the cataract onto the retina surface. If the patient is able to read 20/20 using this direct projection method then their retina MUST be capable of actually SEEING at least 20/20. The "pinhole PAM" technique is similar (and what I use in my office). We have our patients read a brightly illuminated near card in the dark while looking through a pinhole occluder. The pinhole device eliminates any refractive error and the bright letters are "projected" into their eye for the retina to attempt to see. If a patient has an extremely bad cataract, we can't check vision using these techniques, since their eye may only be able to see light versus dark. In such cases, after performing a B-scan ultrasound to rule out retinal detachment and tumors, we check whether the patient can distinguish colored light. I'll put a red or blue eye drop cap over my penlight and ask whether the patient can tell what color light is striking the eye. I also test for "projection," shining a penlight into the eye from different directions. If a patient can't even tell me color or the direction a light is coming from, this bodes poorly for their overall visual potential after surgery. Finally, contrast sensitivity (the detection of subtle differences in gray) is rarely checked. I personally haven't measured contrast sensitivity in years. This technique is more useful for measuring subtle optic nerve dysfunction in conditions like optic neuritis.

12. A capsulorhexis is:
A. a hole created in the capsule
B. the removal of cortical debris from the capsule
C. a loss of zonular support at the edge of the capsule
D. a "run out" of the capsular opening

The correct answer is (a). During normal cataract surgery, we create a capsulorhexis, or "hole," though the front of the cataract capsule. This allows phacoemulsification - removal of the nucleus and cortical debris inside. This capsulorhexis "hole" is not always easy to create, as it involves piercing through clear anterior capsule, grasping this thin tissue with microforceps, and tearing a round hole of the appropriate size (and praying that the patient doesn't cough, sneeze, or turn their head suddenly). Everyone's capsule reacts differently - with bulky cataracts, the hole/tear can "run out" in the wrong direction toward the outer edge of the lens. This run out can even extend around the back surface of the cataract. This is a significant problem, often resulting in a dropped nucleus and a challenging implant insertion.

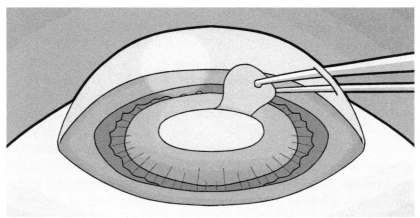

A capsulorhexis is a hole created in the anterior capsule so that the inner layers of the cataract can be removed.

13. PCO are removed:
A. surgically
B. with a laser
C. with a hammer
D. EDTA chelation

The correct answer is (b). A PCO is a posterior capsular opacification or "after cataract." This is an opacity that forms months or years after a normal eye surgery. Residual cells are left in the "bag" (capsule) that proliferate along the back surface of the capsule and create blur. This opacity is very common, occuring in up to 30% of patients following surgery. Fortunately, a PCO is easy to fix: a YAG laser can be utilized to blast a hole through the center of the posterior capsule. It's generally best to wait a few months after cataract surgery before creating this hole, as you don't want any chance that the implant will fall through into the vitreous cavity. I'm not aware of any eye procedures requiring a hammer, though oculoplastic surgeons use some hardcore trocar bone-crunchers when performing DCR drainage surgery into the nose. EDTA chelation is used to help break apart calcium deposits that form on the surface of sick eyes with band keratopathy: the eye is anesthetized and soaked with EDTA to soften the calcium, which is then scraped off the cornea with a scalpel.

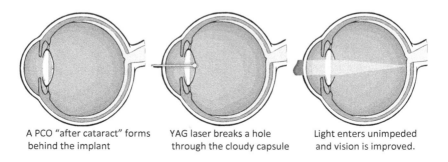

A PCO "after cataract" forms behind the implant

YAG laser breaks a hole through the cloudy capsule

Light enters unimpeded and vision is improved.

14. All of the following can cause a cataract, <u>except</u>:
A. diabetes
B. trauma
C. corticosteroids
D. macular degeneration

The correct answer is (d). While both macular degeneration and cataracts are common as we age, one doesn't cause the other. Diabetes and steroids can certainly cause premature cataract formation, especially PSC cataracts at the back of the lens. Trauma

CHAPTER 2: CATARACT & LENS

can also cause a cataract - either immediately, if the outer cortex has been punctured, or years later. Traumatic cataracts are higher risk, as they may be dense and are sometimes associated with zonular weakness or loss.

15. After cataract surgery, cataracts come back:
A. rarely
B. never ever
C. with incomplete removal of cortex
D. often

The answer is (b). Once a cataract is gone, it can't come back. Many people will develop an "after cataract," or PCO (posterior capsular opacification). This is a clouding of the posterior capsule behind the implant that is easily cleared by using a YAG laser. The cataract itself can't really come back, though, short of divine intervention.

16. The most common cause of cataract is:
A. age
B. genetic predisposition
C. steroid use
D. smoking

The answer here is (a). Cataracts become extremely common as we age. In fact, cataract surgery is the second most common surgery in the United States (right behind circumcision). Oral steroids, chemotherapy, radiation, and smoking are all associated with formation of cataracts. Some people may have a genetic predisposition to early cataract formation and cataracts are associated with a number of genetic disorders.

17. All of the following are types of cataracts, <u>except</u> for:
A. nucular
B. posterior subcapsular
C. cortical
D. Christmas tree

The answer is (a). The most common cataracts we see are <u>nuclear</u> (check that spelling) and cortical. Nuclear cataracts occur in the central nucleus of the lens and look like a yellow or brownish tint to the central lens. Cortical cataracts appear as white, spoke-like stripes coming in from the periphery. Posterior subcapsular cataracts (PSC) look like white sand or breadcrumbs on the back of the lens and are more common in younger people with diabetes or patients taking oral steroids. A "Christmas tree" cataract is one that has the appearance of prismatic shards of glass or the tinsel used to decorate Christmas trees. They are rare and are associated with myotonic dystrophy, though I sometimes see them in patients with no genetic issues.

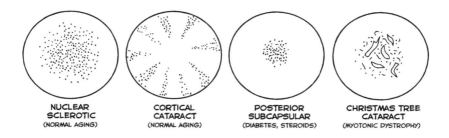

NUCLEAR SCLEROTIC (NORMAL AGING) | CORTICAL CATARACT (NORMAL AGING) | POSTERIOR SUBCAPSULAR (DIABETES, STEROIDS) | CHRISTMAS TREE CATARACT (MYOTONIC DYSTROPHY)

18. Viscoelastics are used in cataract surgery to:
A. facilitate nuclear fragment removal
B. rotate the lens-iris diaphragm forward
C. dampen phacoemulsification energy
D. hydrodissect the lens

The best answer is (c). Viscoelastics are gels containing sodium hyaluronate. They are thick with a consistency of hair gel and injected into the anterior chamber during cataract surgery to keep the anterior chamber from "deflating" as we work on the cataract. They also coat the inside surface of the cornea with a layer of "slime" and help protect the endothelium from vibration/heat energy from the phacoemulsification tip (and from nuclear fragments bouncing around in the AC). These gels do NOT help with nuclear fragment removal, however. If anything, the gels make the cleanup of small pieces of nucleus *more* problematic as the little pieces can wedge themselves in the angle where we can't see them. Hydrodissection is the technique of injecting fluid into the cataract to "dissect" or to separate the outer capsule from the inner cortex/nucleus with water. This facilitates rotation and removal of the inner layers of the cataract. Initial hydrodissection is always done with saline fluid as viscoelastics are too thick.

19. All of the following are techniques for breaking up a cataract, <u>except</u>:
A. divide and conquer
B. stand and deliver
C. stop and chop
D. horizontal chop

The correct answer is (b). There are many methods for breaking up a cataract using the phacoemulsification tip. Most residents learn the standard divide and conquer technique. This involves grooving two trenches in the nucleus like an X or cross. The cataract is then broken into four different quadrants and each is removed individually. Other techniques use a "chopping motion." For example, with the horizontal chop, the phacoemulsification probe is embedded into the cataract like a lollipop. After this, a small metal wand (usually the Connor wand) is slipped around one edge of the nucleus and the two instruments are brought together. This effectively breaks the cataract into two pieces without using energy to create a trench first. Stand and Deliver was a movie from the '80s about an inner-city school teacher.

20. An advancing cataract may cause all of the following, except:
A. becoming more nearsighted
B. becoming more farsighted
C. decreasing dependence on glasses
D. increased accommodation

The best answer here is (d). As a cataract develops, it typically make the lens larger and denser. This usually creates a myopic shift (nearsightedness) as the powerful cataract is too strong, focusing images in the vitreous cavity instead of on the retina. Occasionally, we'll see a hyperopic (farsighted) shift. Refractive shifts are often a sign that a cataract is beginning to worsen. For some, this refractive change occurs in a "good direction," and they happily find themselves less dependant on their old glasses. Their eyes haven't become "better," just changing. This phenomenon is sometimes called "second sight." Accommodation is the ability of the lens to change shape, usually in an attempt to read near objects. Cataracts don't improve lens flexibility, so cataracts never help with accommodation.

21. Early cataracts are associated with the following, except:
A. diabetes
B. amiodarone
C. prednisone
D. radiation

The best answer is (b). The main cause of cataracts is age, but for young people, they can occur from diabetes, steroid use, and radiation (such as from cancer treatment). Amiodarone is an antiarrhythmic heart medication that can cause corneal deposits called "verticillata." These deposits are common, and patients are always amazed when I ask them (after looking at their eyes) if they take this medication.

CHAPTER 2: CATARACT & LENS

22. Cataracts cause the following symptoms, <u>except</u>:
A. glare
B. halos
C. loss of contrast
D. increased tearing

The best answer is (d). Cataracts occur INSIDE the eye and cause vision loss. They don't cause tearing or eye pain. This is important to emphasize to your patient before eye surgery, as people will associate tearing with their cataract and be quite upset with you when the epiphora continues after surgery.

23. What cataract causes the <u>least</u> vision problems:
A. mature
B. senile
C. hypermature
D. Morgagnian

The correct answer is (b). A senile cataract is just a regular cataract that occurs from age. The word "senile" is often used in medicine to describe changes secondary to aging - it is not meant to imply "decrepit" or "inferior." For example, people can have a senile ptosis or senile ectropion of the eyelids that occurs from eyelid laxity with age. A "mature" cataract usually refers to a ripe or hard cataract (possibly white in color) that is very dense and ready for cataract surgery. The term "hypermature" or "Morgagnian" is used to describe an ultra-dense cataract that has been ignored for years. These cataracts are often so bad that the cortex has liquefied into a white, milky fluid while the nucleus has hardened into a brown nut that has sunk to the bottom of the capsular bag. Hypermature cataracts can sometimes cause inflammation in the eye if the cortical "milk" leaks into the aqueous fluid.

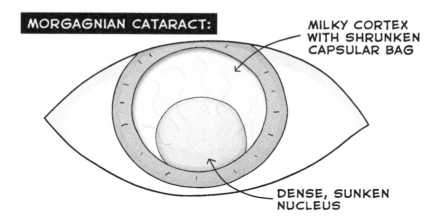

24. When removing a cataract, <u>where</u> is it possible to enter the eye?
A. clear cornea
B. sclera
C. pars plana
D. all of the above

The correct answer is actually (d). Most modern cataract surgery is performed as a "clear cornea" microincision through the cornea. However, a cataract incision can also be made through the white sclera ... the surgeon then tunnels the incision forward into the clear cornea before entering the anterior chamber. These "scleral tunnels" are usually reserved for complicated cases where a larger incision is anticipated, because large scleral incisions will cause less corneal edema and distortion. Rarely, a retina doctor will remove a cataract from "behind" by entering the eye posteriorly through the "pars plana." This might be done after a dislocated or traumatic cataract, where the lens can't be phacoemulsified or "grabbed" from the front.

CHAPTER 2: CATARACT & LENS

25. A retrobulbar block affects all of the nerves, <u>except</u>:
A. CN 2
B. CN 3
C. CN 4
D. CN 6

The correct answer is (c). A retrobulbar block is an anesthesia method where lidocaine is injected into the muscle cone behind the eye. Cranial nerves 3 and 6 run inside this cone, so all of the rectus muscles are paralyzed. The optic nerve (CN2) is also paralyzed. As a result, patients will have dim vision after a block. The 4th cranial nerve, however, runs OUTSIDE the retrobulbar space, along with the circuitous superior oblique muscle, and so is unaffected. After a block, we always ask our patients to look up and down. With a good block, the eye will only rotate a little because the only muscle working is the superior oblique.

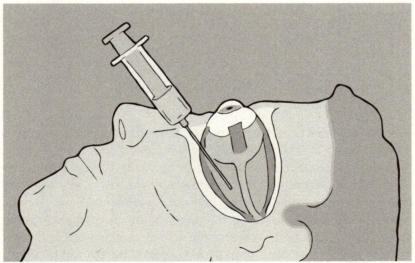

With a retrobulbar block, anesthetic is injected into the "muscle cone" behind the eye.

26. The lens contributes what percentage of the refractive power of the eye?
A. 30%
B. 50%
C. 70%
D. 100%

The best answer is (a). The lens, despite its importance for focusing, only contributes about a third of the overall refractive power of the eyeball. The cornea is actually responsible for most of the refraction of light in our eye.

27. Hyperglycemia can affect the lens by:
A. making it swell
B. making it shrink
C. making it go limp
D. making it excited

The correct answer is (a). The lens is a living tissue that is avascular. It gets its nutrition through glycolysis from sugars in the aqueous fluid. Hyperglycemia can change the metabolism in the lens such that sorbitol is generated and builds up in the lens. This sugar alcohol (also found in sugarless chewing gum) creates an osmotic gradient and pulls water into the lens, making it swell. A swollen lens is too "powerful," focusing images in the vitreous cavity, and causing temporary nearsightedness. This myopic shift may take several weeks to resolve, so we may have our poorly controlled diabetic patients come back for a glasses recheck.

28. Most modern lens implants are:
A. silicone
B. three-piece
C. multifocal
D. aspheric

The best answer is (d). Implant technology has improved over the last few decades. Today, most modern implants are flexible lenses made from a single piece of acrylic plastic. This flexible lens can be folded and inserted through a very small corneal incision. Once inside the eye, the central "optic" unfolds and two "haptic" arms spring out, centering the lens inside the capsule. Older three-piece lenses are still used as their longer haptics (often made of prolene) are helpful with complicated cases or when capsular insufficiencies force you to place the implant in the sulcus (between the capsule and iris). Multifocal lenses, such as the ReSTOR implant from Alcon, have concentric rings that create two focal points and can help patients read without glasses. These multifocal implants have downsides (glare, halos and expense) and aren't used as often as the standard lenses. Most modern implants are aspheric, with the front surface being less steep at the edges - this allows the lens to better match the aspheric cornea and can improve contrast and clarity.

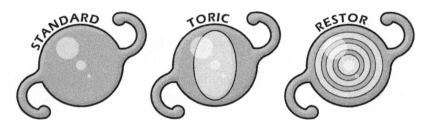

Most patients get a standard monofocal lens. There are more expensive implants available, such as the astigmatism-correcting toric lens and the multifocal ReSTOR lens.

29. What medicine is commonly used intracamerally during cataract surgery?
A. lidocaine
B. tetracaine
C. gentamicin
D. Ancef

The correct answer is (a). The word "intracameral" means within the anterior chamber. We inject preservative-free lidocaine into the anterior chamber during cataract surgery to numb the iris muscle. Care must be given with any injection in the eye as you can't use preservatives here. The cornea endothelium is extremely delicate (we use MPF lidocaine, which stands for methylparaben free). Tetracaine is only available in drop format. Gentamicin is an antibiotic that is used topically. It is contraindicated for intraocular use as it causes retina issues. Ancef is an antibiotic that is commonly used empirically through an IV during surgery. We don't typically use this in routine cataract surgery, but it might be appropriate during an open-globe repair.

30. What is the intermediate layer of the lens called?
A. cortex
B. capsule
C. nucleus
D. epinucleus

The correct answer is (a). The intermediate layer of a cataract is called the cortex. It is clear, and normally has the consistency of Jell-O. During surgery, we create a hole through the capsule to gain access to the inner layers. The nucleus is removed via phacoemulsification. The residual cortex is then stripped out in pieces - like sucking out Jell-O with a straw. Residual cortex can cause opacities and inflammation after surgery, so we try to clean it up and polish the capsular bag as clear we can before inserting the new implant.

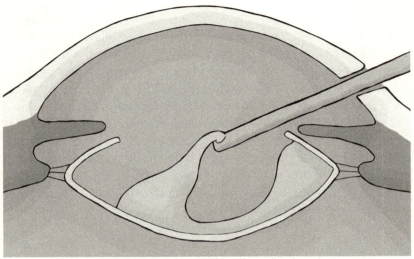

The intermediate cortex is removed, like sucking Jell-O through a straw.

31. Trypan blue (Visionblue) is used to stain:
A. vitreous
B. capsule
C. cortex
D. cornea

The correct answer is (b). Visionblue is a blue dye that is sometimes used during cataract surgery to stain the surface of the lens capsule. During cataract surgery, we create a round hole through the clear capsule to access the inner layers of the cataract. This hole is called a capsulorhexis and its creation is one of the hardest steps of cataract surgery. The capsule is thin like cellophane and extremely hard to see in patients with dense cataracts. It is much easier to see the capsule when it's stained blue, however. Trypan blue makes the surgery safer with less chance of a capsule run-out during construction.

32. BAT testing is primarily used to detect:
A. macular degeneration
B. dry eye
C. cataracts
D. rabies

The best answer here is (c). The brightness acuity test is used to detect glare sensitivity, and is a common test used when checking for cataracts. Opacities in the lens cause light to scatter, resulting in glare at night. The BAT test attempts to quantify this blur by shooting light into the eye while the patient reads the eye chart. Macular degeneration usually creates problems with dark adaptation. After shining a light in a patient's eyes, patients may take a long time (minutes) to adapt to dim lighting enough to read the eye chart. Dry eye has no effect on glare, though these patients are sensitive to sunlight. Bats can carry rabies, but we don't check for that during an eye exam.

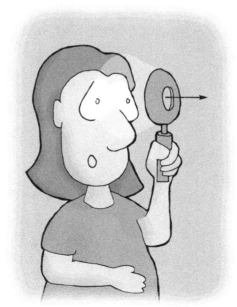

The BAT (brightness acuity test) device. We often just recheck our patient's vision while shining a penlight in their eye.

33. What medicines are associated with floppy iris syndrome (FIS)?
A. hypertensive medicine
B. urinary medication
C. cholesterol medication
D. hormone medication

The correct answer is (b). The alpha-blocking urinary medications like Flomax (tamsulosin) relax smooth muscle in the bladder to help with urination. However, these medications also relax the smooth muscle that makes up the iris, making it floppy. During cataract surgery, the iris can be so floppy that it prolapses out of the incision, subsequently making the surgery quite difficult. Iris is extremely difficult to handle. Under the microscope, it has the consistency of wet tissue paper, tearing easily with manipulation. We deal with floppy iris by using iris hooks or a Malyugin ring to hold the iris down. We also use generous amounts of viscoelastic gels during the case to push the iris out of the incisions. Safety sutures may need to be placed in the corneal incisions after surgery to keep the iris from prolapsing or sticking in the incision tunnel. Oddly, the floppy iris effect lasts for months or years after cessation of the oral medication.

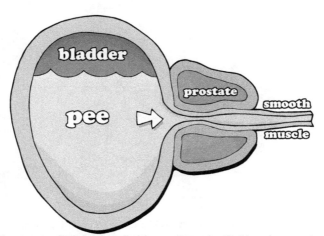

The same medications that relax the prostate, relax the iris and can create "floppy iris syndrome" during surgery.

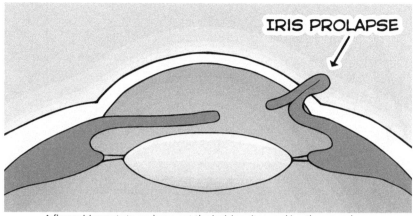

A floppy iris wants to prolapse out the incision sites, making the procedure much more difficult.

34. A Malyugin ring is used in surgery to help with:
A. zonular dehiscence
B. broken capsule
C. small pupils
D. shallow chamber

The best answer is (c). The Malyugin ring is a collapsible spring made of plastic that can be injected into the eye to dilate the pupil. This is extremely helpful with poorly dilating patients and those with floppy iris syndrome, as the ring keeps the iris in place. The other answers are incorrect, but they do bring up a few learning points. Zonular dehiscence occurs when the zonular "springs" that suspend the capsule begin to break. If enough zonules break, the entire lens can dislocate into the vitreous cavity. To decrease zonular trauma, we occasionally place a capsular tension ring inside the capsule. This ring expands and keeps the edge of the capsule round while manipulating the rest of the cataract. By maintaining the proper anatomy, no more zonular springs will snap off (hopefully). A broken posterior capsule is the most common cataract complication. This is repaired with an anterior vitrectomy to remove any vitreous strands that have prolapsed up into the anterior chamber.

CHAPTER 2: CATARACT & LENS

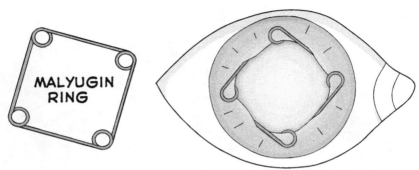

The Malyugin ring is awesome ... much faster and less traumatic then iris hooks.

CHAPTER 3
CORNEA

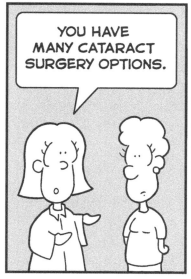
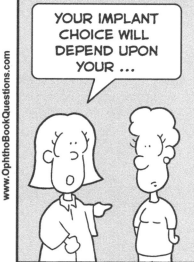
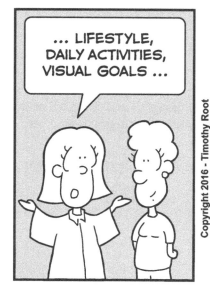
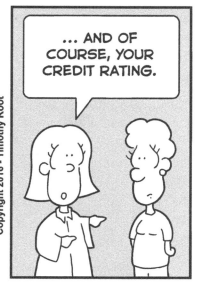

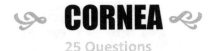

CORNEA
25 Questions

1. The cornea receives nutrition via all, <u>except</u>:
A. tear film
B. aqueous
C. limbal vessels
D. canal of Schlemm

The correct answer is (d). The cornea, like the lens, is an avascular structure without any blood vessels in it, except at the limbal edge. It receives most of its nutrition and oxygen from the tear film on the outside and the aqueous fluid on the inside. The canal of Schlemm is the venous drainage located behind the trabecular meshwork where aqueous is absorbed back into the bloodstream.

2. To fix nearsightedness with a laser, the cornea must be:
A. flattened
B. steepened
C. strengthened
D. stiffened

The correct answer is (a). People who are nearsighted have large, powerful eyes. Their refractive system is so strong that images focus in the vitreous gel, in front of the retina. To push the image back onto the retina, the cornea must be weakened and, therefore, flattened as well. This can be accomplished with an excimer laser during LASIK or PRK by ablating away central corneal tissue.

3. Which refractive surgery uses lasers but no flap?
A. PRK
B. RK
C. LASIK
D. LASEK

The correct answer is (a). PRK is the procedure where the laser is applied directly to the front of the cornea. The surface of the epithelium is scraped off prior to applying the laser treatment, but no flap is created and the epithelium quickly regrows back over the new surface. LASIK surgery involves cutting a flap through the stroma and applying the laser to the exposed stromal bed. This is advantageous due to quicker healing time and less discomfort. LASEK is similar to PRK, but a thin "epithelial flap" is created and pushed back into place after laser treatment to speed abrasion healing. RK is an older surgery that involves diamond knives to cut spoke-like cuts in the cornea to reshape it.

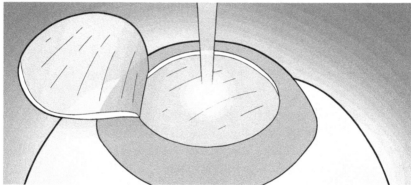

With LASIK, a flap is made in the cornea.

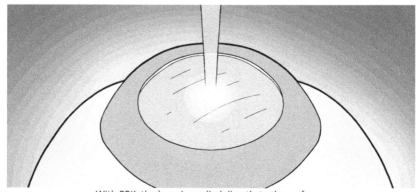

With PRK, the laser is applied directly to the surface.

CHAPTER 3: CORNEA

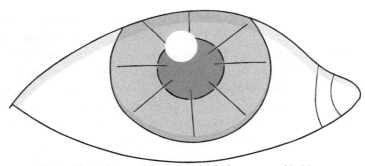

RK is an older technique that uses partial thickness corneal incisions.

4. Which layer of the cornea is deepest?
A. stroma
B. endothelium
C. Bowman's layer
D. Descemet's layer

The correct answer is (b). The endothelium on the inside of the cornea is the "deepest" followed by Descemet's membrane. If you need help remembering the location of Descemet's layer compared to Bowman's layer, just remember that <u>D</u>escemet's is <u>d</u>eep.

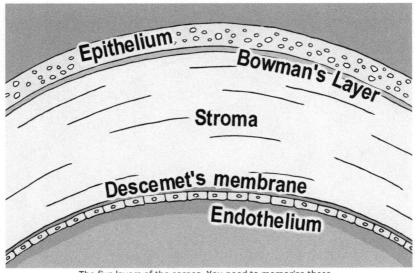

The five layers of the cornea. You need to memorize these.

5. What layer of the cornea is ablated with LASIK surgery?
A. epithelium
B. Bowman's layer
C. stroma
D. Descemet's layer

The correct answer is (c). With LASIK surgery, a flap is created through the anterior stroma and lifted. The laser is then applied directly to the stromal bed underneath to change the shape of the cornea. The benefit to this approach is quicker healing as the surface epithelium is left mostly intact.

6. Patients with Fuchs' dystrophy may exhibit all of the following, <u>except</u> for:
A. polymegathism
B. pleomorphism
C. polydactyly
D. guttae

The correct answer is (c). Fuchs' dystrophy is a condition where people are born with less endothelial cells than normal. This is significant as these cells act as "pump" cells to keep the cornea dry and clear. These cells don't replicate or regenerate. As the cells die, whether through natural attrition or during eye surgery, the remaining cells enlarge (polymegathism) and vary their shape (pleomorphism). This can be seen using direct specular microscopy. Guttae (sometimes called "guttata") are little bumps or divots seen with the slit-lamp microscope on the back surface of the cornea. It is the most common finding with Fuchs'. Polydactyly is when you have extra fingers and is unrelated to Fuchs'.

CHAPTER 3: CORNEA

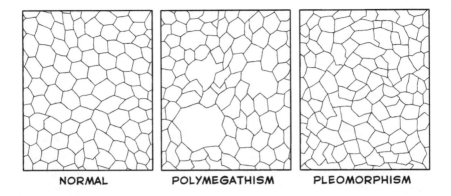

7. Contact lens "overwear" can cause all, <u>except</u>:
A. new blood vessels
B. eyelid bumps
C. micro-ulcers
D. conjunctival pigmentation

The best answer is (d). Contact lens use has some obvious risks, especially infectious ulcers from bacteria like pseudomonas. In addition, some people can develop an allergic/sensitivity reaction called GPC (giant papillary conjunctivitis) where giant bumps form on the underside of the upper eyelid. Finally, contact lenses decrease the amount of oxygen to the cornea, which can cause new blood vessels or a "panus" to form along the limbus (the outer edge of the cornea). Pigmentation is usually from normal melanin (we see harmless "racial melanosis" in darker skinned patients) or potential malignancy.

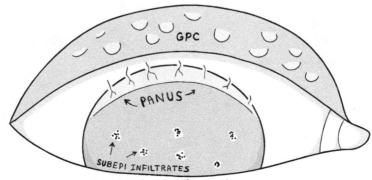

Some complications of contact lens overwear

9. The cornea is steepest:
A. mid-peripherally
B. at the limbus
C. centrally
D. where it is thickest

The best answer is (c). The cornea is generally steepest in the middle and flattens out as it approaches the limbal edge. The cornea is also thinner in the middle, averaging around 540 microns by pachymetry measurements. The steepness variability means that the cornea isn't a "perfect" lens - it contains a certain amount of "spherical aberration." Fortunately, most of this aberration is balanced by the lens, which is flattest in the middle. "Ectatic" disorders like keratoconus don't follow this rule and may show maximal corneal steepness in a more inferior location.

10. PK (penetrating keratoplasty) is a fancy way to describe:
A. full-thickness corneal laceration repair
B. corneal resurfacing
C. corneal transplant
D. deep corneal laser treatment

The correct answer is (c). A PK is another way of saying corneal transplant. It is referred to as "penetrating" to imply that the graft is a full thickness procedure. A lamellar keratoplasty implies that only part of the cornea (not full thickness) has been replaced.

11. An appropriate treatment for a contact-lens-related ulcer on the cornea might include:
A. maxitrol
B. erythromycin
C. tobramycin
D. proparacaine

CHAPTER 3: CORNEA

The best answer is (c). Infections from contact lens tend to be rapid and aggressive antibiotic coverage is recommended. Tobramycin has decent coverage for pseudomonas infection, as do fluoroquinolone drops like ciprofloxacin and gatifloxacin. Maxitrol is a trade name for a cheap combination drop containing neomycin, polymyxin and dexamethasone steroid. A steroid drop like this is *never* a good idea with corneal infections: bacteria (and viruses and fungi) love steroids and will replicate even faster. Proparacaine is the numbing eye drop used in the office. While good for anesthesia, it is toxic to the cornea when used repeatedly and will keep the cornea from healing. Never prescribe your patient a numbing drop. Finally, erythromycin ointment is a great general use antibiotic appropriate for minor infections, but you need something stronger with corneal ulcers.

12. A recurrent corneal erosion involves poor adhesion between:
A. endothelium and epithelium
B. epithelium and Descemet's layer
C. epithelium and Bowman's layer
D. endothelium and Descemet's layer

The answer here is (c). A recurrent corneal erosion occurs after a corneal abrasion, when the epithelium doesn't stick down well to the underlying Bowman's layer. The epithelium can reopen with minor insults and cause recurring corneal abrasions. Corneal erosions typically occur after minor lacerations. We often see this amoung parents who have been scratched by a baby's fingernail or hit in the eye with a toy.

13. Treatments for a recurrent corneal erosion includes the following, except:
A. ointment
B. stromal puncture
C. corneal polishing
D. hypoosmotic drops

The correct answer here is (d). Recurring erosions are tricky to treat as the epithelium does not want to stick down to the eye. Minor insults, such as opening the eyes in the morning, can reopen the loose flap of tissue. Most doctors start with conservative measures such as rewetting drops, ointments, and bandage contact lens. If this doesn't work, a hyperosmotic drop like Muro 128 may help suck water out of the cornea and hold the skin in place. If these methods aren't working, a small bent needle can be used to puncture divots in the cornea stroma. This provides an area for epithelium to grow into, helping better anchor it. This may create a small scar, however, and may not be appropriate if the erosion is located in the central cornea. Corneal polishing with a spinning burr may smooth the underlying stroma and allow better epithelial adhesion.

14. An appropriate prescribed analgesic for a corneal abrasion would be:
A. tetracaine
B. proparacaine
C. lidocaine
D. polyvinyl alcohol

The correct answer would be (d). It is *never* good to use anesthetic eye drops with a corneal abrasion, except in the office to facilitate the eye exam. These medications are toxic to the cornea and will delay healing. The medicines will keep the cornea epithelium from growing and can turn an otherwise uncomplicated abrasion into a non-healing ulcer. It's rare, but some of the worse corneas I've seen were from people who were inadvertently given (or stole) a bottle of tetracaine. The ER uses tetracaine and I've had patients grab the bottle upon discharge and use it every fifteen minutes because their "eye hurt." You must confiscate these bottles from the patient and use oral analgesics if necessary. Polyvinyl alcohol, despite the odd name, is a thickening agent/lubricant used in some artificial tears.

CHAPTER 3: CORNEA

15. A patient develops a large cornea abrasion after poking himself in the eye with an artificial Christmas tree. Appropriate treatments include all, <u>except</u>:
A. patching for 48 hours
B. contact lens
C. antibiotic ointment
D. oral analgesics

The best answer is (a). Patching is an acceptable treatment for treating a large, painful corneal abrasion, but it must be done with extreme caution. Don't patch an eye at risk for infection (contact lens wearers or "dirty" wounds), since bacteria like warm, dark places. Also, don't patch for more than 24 hours. The other choices are all appropriate, though I usually reserve "bandage" contact lenses for people with slow-healing abrasions or if they have a lot of pain and don't want their eye patched. Oral analgesics are a good idea as topical anesthesia will delay healing.

16. Treatment for Fuchs' may involve all, <u>except</u>:
A. sodium bicarbonate
B. salty ointments
C. corneal transplant
D. hyperosmotic drops

The correct answer is (a). Fuchs' dystrophy is a common corneal condition where a person is born with less endothelial pump cells than normal. This causes their cornea to become too wet and cloudy, especially in the morning. Initial treatment is usually a hyperosmotic drop called Muro 128. This eye drop has a high concentration of sodium chloride that osmotically pulls some of the excess water from the cornea. It is available in both liquid and ointment form. Recalcitrant Fuchs' may require a corneal transplant to replace the endothelium - this used to be performed as a full-thickness PK but is now performed as a partial thickness DSEK procedure. Sodium bicarbonate is the active ingredient in baking soda (and Alka-Seltzer), and is sometimes used clinically via IV for acidosis. It is not used in the eye.

17. RK surgery involves:
A. excimer laser
B. femtosecond laser
C. sharp knives
D. radio cautery

The correct answer is (c). RK (radial keratotomy) is an older refractive surgery where diamond knives were used to create radial incisions in the cornea. This helped flatten the cornea and correct nearsightedness by weakening the overall focal power of the eye. Excimer laser is used with LASIK and PRK surgery to ablate corneal tissue. The femtosecond laser (Intralase) is used to create cuts and flaps during refractive surgery. We also use a femtosecond laser with "laser cataract surgery" to create corneal incisions, capsulorhexis, and help break up the nucleus.

18. Corneal thickness is relevant to all, except:
A. glaucoma
B. endothelial dystrophy
C. epithelial dystrophy
D. refractive surgery

The best answer is (c). Corneal thickness is relevant to glaucoma as it affects pressure readings during applanation tonometry. Endothelial dystrophies, such as Fuchs' dystrophy, result in thicker corneas because of fluid buildup in the corneal stroma. The thickness of the cornea is also important in refractive surgery: LASIK and PRK are contraindicated if the cornea is too thin to treat. The most common epithelial dystrophy is called EBMD (epithelial basement membrane dystrophy), which is commonly known as "map-dot-fingerprint" dystrophy. This condition is quite common, and increases the chance of corneal abrasion from a loosely adherent epithelial layer on the surface of the eye. Corneal thickness is irrelevant to epithelial problems.

19. All of the following dyes are commonly used on the cornea, except for:
A. fluorescein salt
B. lissamine green
C rose bengal
D. indocyanine green

The correct answer is (d). Fluorescein is the dye we use in clinic to detect corneal abrasions and is used during applanation tonometry. Both rose bengal and lissamine green can be used during the slit-lamp exam as they stain irritated and damaged cells. This is useful for detecting patterns of dry eye such as SLK (found with thyroid disease). I rarely bother with these dyes, but they are a favorite for many cornea and "dry eye" specialists. Rose bengal is the better known of the two, but it is cytotoxic and can sting. Lissamine green is a harmless food additive that seems to work just as well and is better tolerated. The green color is also easier to see. Indocyanine green is not used on the ocular surface but injected into the arm during an ICG angiogram of the deep retina and choroid.

20. Common conditions requiring a cornea transplant include all, except:
A. Fuchs' dystrophy
B. herpetic infection
C. arcus senilis
D. keratoconus

The correct answer is (c). The most common entities that lead to corneal transplant are intractable edema from Fuchs' dystrophy, scarring from herpetic infection, and irregular astigmatism from keratoconus. Other conditions that might require a transplant include perforating ulcers and trauma. Arcus senilis is a harmless whitening of the peripheral cornea that occurs from age. Arcus is harmless, though it may be associated with high-cholesterol when found in youth and asymmetric carotid disease when found in only one eye. It does not cause vision problems and never requires a transplant.

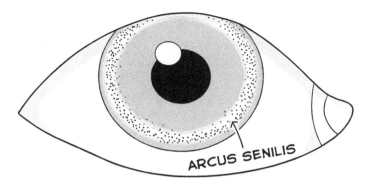

21. Best treatment for a corneal dellen is:
A. lubrication
B. corneal scraping
C. corneal patch graft
D. amniotic membrane

The correct answer is (a). A dellen is a thin area of the cornea that occurs from localized dehydration. This usually occurs along the corneal edge near raised conjunctival lesions. For example, if a patient has a bad subconjunctival hemorrhage (bleeding under the conjunctival skin) a raised hematoma of blood may form. With blinking, the eyelids bounce over this "mountain" of tissue and fail to spread the tear film in the "valley" next to it. Dellen can look impressive! They may make you nervous that the eye will perforate. However, aggressive lubrication with ointments will almost always cause the tissue to rehydrate and look "normal" within a day. Dellen are not an infection, and therefore do not require a scrape biopsy for culture. They rarely perforate, so grafting is not needed. The epithelium is intact, so an amniotic membrane contact is overkill, uncomfortable, and very expensive.

22. All of the following procedures require lasers, except:
A. PRK
B. PK
C. YAG
D. SLT

CHAPTER 3: CORNEA

The best answer is (b). A PK, or penetrating keratoplasty, is a full-thickness corneal transplant. It is performed by using a round cutting blade (a trephine) that is rotated to cut down into the corneal surface. Some cornea doctors have experimented using lasers to cut more precisely through both the host and donor cornea tissue, but this isn't standard. PRK is a refractive laser surgery similar to LASIK, except no flap is created and the laser is applied to the front surface of the eye. A YAG laser can have several uses, but is most commonly used to laser away capsular opacification that has formed on the back of an implant years after cataract surgery. SLT is a glaucoma procedure where the YAG laser is used to stimulate the trabecular meshwork cells to flow better.

23. A growth of conjunctival skin growing over the cornea is:
A. pinguecula
B. pterygium
C. ptolemy
D. pterosaur

The correct answer is (b). A pterygium is a growth of conjunctival skin that crosses over the limbus and onto the cornea. It is very common in people who get a lot of sun exposure (surfers, construction workers) and can be removed if it causes irritation, astigmatism, or looks unsightly. A pinguecula is a similar bump, but only on the conjunctiva. Ptolemy was an ancient scholar and mathematician. The pterosaur is a winged dinosaur and the first flying vertebrate capable of powered flight.

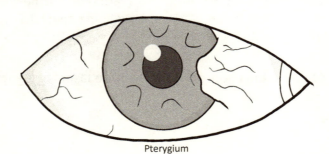
Pterygium

24. A pterygium removal may be facilitated with all, <u>except</u> for:
A. amniotic membrane
B. mitomycin
C. pericardium
D. autograft

The best answer is (c). A pterygium is a flap of conjunctival tissue that has grown over the surface of the cornea. There are many ways to remove a pterygium. The easiest approach is to cut it out, leaving "bare sclera" underneath. Unfortunately, this allows the pterygium to grow back, generally leading to a high recurrence rate. Antimetabolites such as mitomycin have been used, though I've never liked them for this purpose because of the risk for scleral melt. The most definitive treatment is with an "autograft." After the pterygium is removed, a small piece of conjunctiva from under the eyelid is harvested and sewn over the sclera where the pterygium was first located. This radically decreases regrowth, but the surgery is tedious as it is difficult to sew conjunctiva. Amniotic membrane grafts have been used, though I've had mixed results. Pericardium isn't used for pterygium surgery, but it is used during glaucoma tube-shunt surgery. Sterilized pericardium, also known as Tutoplast, can be cut with scissors and sewn over a tube, decreasing the chance that the tube will erode up through the conjunctiva and become exposed to air.

25. Band keratopathy is composed of:
A. iron
B. immune deposits
C. calcium
D. rock stars

The best answer is (c). Band keratopathy is calcium that forms on the surface of the cornea in sick eyes. Patients with chronic inflammation (uveitis), end-stage glaucoma, or retinal detachments can develop changes in the metabolism in the eye. The pH of their tear film may change, resulting in calcium precipitates that stick to the corneal surface. This calcium can further decrease vision and cause pain from repeated corneal abrasions. Treatment is with EDTA chelation solution applied to the cornea surface, followed by scraping the calcium off with a curved scalpel blade. Ouch! The other answers are incorrect, however, a thin iron line on the cornea is common in people with chronic dry eye.

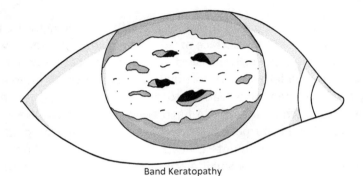

Band Keratopathy

CHAPTER 4
GENERAL

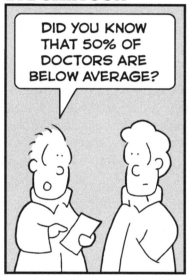
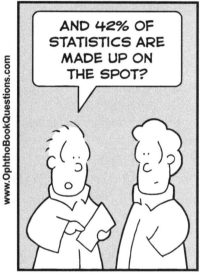
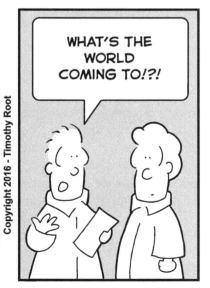

GENERAL

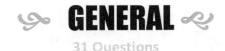

31 Questions

1. Protrusion of the eye from thyroid eye disease is commonly called:
A. exophthalmos
B. enophthalmos
C. proptosis
D. ptosis

The best answer is (a). Both proptosis and exophthalmos are terms used to describe an eye that is bulging out from the eye socket. Exophthalmos, however, is usually reserved for bulging that occurs from thyroid disorder (Graves' disease). Enophthalmos is an eye that has shrunken into the orbit (usually after an orbital wall fracture) and ptosis is a droopy eyelid.

2. If a patient has both cataracts and macular degeneration affecting vision, a good test to differentiate the major visual culprit is:
A. contrast sensitivity
B. BAT testing
C. PAM testing
D. RAT testing

The best answer is (c). When our cataract patients have coexisting retinal pathology, it is often hard to determine how much of their vision is affected by the cataract itself. One technique we use is the PAM (potential acuity meter). This gadget projects an image onto the retina. If we measure good vision using the PAM, then we know that the retina must be capable of good vision as well. BAT (brightness acuity test) measures the effects of glare on vision. While glare usually occurs from cataract, the BAT test is somewhat nonspecific. Contrast sensitivity is rarely measured, and not terribly helpful. RAT testing is performed by restaurant health inspectors.

3. Heterochromia refers to:
A. ocular mosaicism
B. asymmetric color vision
C. different colored irises
D. red-green color blindness

The correct answer is (c). Heterochromia is when the iris color looks different between the eyes. While common in dogs, it is much less common in humans. There are a few odd causes of heterochromia, such as intraocular iron body and congenital Horner's syndrome, but most cases are congenital. Asymmetric color vision implies dysfunction of the optic nerve, such as that seen from optic neuritis (multiple sclerosis). Red-green color blindness is extremely common in men.

4. PERRLA stands for:
A. pupils equally round and reactive to light and accommodation
B. pupils equally round and reactive to light and anisocoric
C. pupils ears and respirations really like-able
D. a fancy lingerie store

The correct answer is (a). PERRLA is a common eye abbreviation used outside of ophthalmology. We don't typically use this phrase in ophthalmology, as our notes are more detailed. Anisocoria is when the pupil size is asymmetric. La Perla is a fancy lingerie store.

5. Marcus Gunn pupil is caused by:
A. projectile sclopteria
B. roman legionella
C. afferent nerve deficiency
D. ciliary nerve damage

The correct answer is (c). A Marcus Gunn pupil is simply an afferent pupil defect (APD). Projectile sclopteria is shockwave damage to the eye as a bullet passes nearby. Legionella is a water-born bacteria that is associated with standing water and air-conditioning systems. It was discovered in 1976 at an American Legion (war veteran organization) meeting in Philadelphia when the bacteria colonized a hotel air-condition system and killed 29 attendees. The ciliary nerve travels behind the eye and carries parasympathetic input to the iris and ciliary body. When damaged, the pupil may dilate (can't constrict) - this is called an Adie's pupil.

6. The movement of an eye by itself, irrespective of the other eye, is often described as a:
A. duction
B. version
C. unasyn
D. torsion

The correct answer is (a). A duction describes the movement of an eye in the cardinal directions, while versions are how the eyes move relative to each other (convergence and divergence). Torsion is how the eye rotates and Unasyn is an IV antibiotic containing ampicillin/sulbactam.

7. An Argyll Robertson pupil is caused by:
A. crocodiles
B. textile allergy
C. STD
D. nerve compression

The correct answer is (c). The Argyll Robertson pupil is caused by neurosyphilis nerve damage. They are small pupils that accommodate (constrict with reading) but weirdly don't react to light. They are sometimes described as the "prostitute's pupil," because prostitutes are known to "accommodate" a customer but don't tend to "react" with true passion. Argyle sweaters have that classic diamond pattern on the front and aren't related to pupil damage (or crocodiles). Nerve compression would cause an APD (afferent pupillary defect, or "Marcus Gunn") pupil.

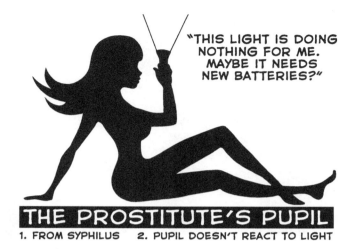

8. Abnormal pupil response is often documented as:
A. PEARL
B. RAPD
C. PERRLA
D. RAPID

The correct answer is (b). A pupil deficiency or APD (afferent pupil defect) is detected in relation to the <u>other</u> eye during the swinging light test. Therefore, we document this as an RAPD (<u>relative</u> afferent pupil defect). The other abbreviations aren't used in ophthalmology.

9. A fixed non-moving pupil may be caused by everything <u>except</u>:
A. glaucoma
B. uveitis
C. trauma
D. retinal detachment

The best answer is (d). Retinal detachment rarely causes pupil problems. If the detachment is large, the patient can develop an APD in the eye, but the pupil still moves normally when you shine light in the <u>other</u> eye via the consensual response. Acute glaucoma can make the pupil appear stuck in a mid-peripheral position as the lens is shoved forward into the back of the iris. Uveitis can cause iris synechia (adhesions) to form, sticking the pupil margin down to the lens underneath. Trauma may also cause dilation if the iris is damaged.

10. What ocular history should you ask your patient about?
A. prior eye surgeries
B. history of cataract surgery
C. history of eye laser procedure
D. all of the above

The correct answer is (d). This is a very easy question, I will admit. It does bring forward an important point, however. Cataract surgery and LASIK have become so commonplace now, that many patients won't mention them to you during a casual questioning. Many people don't think of their eye procedure as a "surgery," so we must ask them directly about cataracts and laser refractive surgery.

11. What is the least important pertinent family eye history?
A. blindness
B. open-angle glaucoma
C. closed-angle glaucoma
D. cataract

The correct answer is (d). Cataract formation is a normal aging change that occurs with everyone to some degree. With rare exceptions, cataracts aren't hereditary and are rarely associated with inheritable syndromes. It is important to ask about familial blindness, however, as this can sometimes elicit a history of retinitis pigmentosa. Glaucoma (especially acute "closed-angle" glaucoma) is heritable and an important risk factor to know about.

12. Which review of systems is least important to an eye doctor treating glaucoma?
A. tooth extraction
B. bradycardia
C. emphysema
D. asthma

The correct answer is (a). While a tooth extraction could cause an infected abscess which could, in theory, track up to the orbit ... this is very unlikely. However, glaucoma is common and one of the most popular treatments is the beta-blocker medication timolol. This drug is administered topically and can absorb through the nose to cause systemic side effects. Beta-blockers can cause bronchospasm and slow the heart rate. You might want to avoid this medicine in patients with breathing issues or heart problems.

13. What systemic allergy is the most important to an eye doctor?
A. sulfa allergy
B. penicillin allergy
C. latex allergy
D. none of the above

The best answer is (a). The most important allergy for an eye doctor is sulfa because an entire class of glaucoma drops (the carbonic anhydrase inhibitors) are sulfa-based. Penicillin allergy isn't as critical as most of the eye drop antibiotics used are either aminoglycosides (tobramycin) or fluoroquinolones (ciprofloxacin, gatifloxacin) with low cross-reactivity. Latex allergy is important during surgery and easily dealt with by using different gloves/instrumentation.

14. Captain Kirk from Star Trek wore reading glasses because:
A. they were given to him by Spock
B. he was allergic to Retinax 5
C. they were his father's spectacles
D. chicks dig scars and glasses

CHAPTER 4: GENERAL

The correct answer is (b). In the original Star Trek: The Wrath of Khan, Kirk (played by William Shatner) is given a set of reading glasses by Doctor McCoy. Kirk suffers from presbyopia as he was one of the few people allergic to Retinax 5.

15. Kenalog (triamcinolone) steroid is used with the eye for all, except:
A. glaucoma
B. uveitis
C. post operative edema
D. anterior vitrectomy

The best answer is (a). Steroids are NOT used with glaucoma as many people are "steroid responders" and will develop high eye pressures on steroids (topical or oral). Steroids are good for inflammation, and occasionally an injection of kenalog steroid is required for treating uveitis or retinal edema if topical steroid drops aren't doing the job. The medicine is sometimes used during complicated cataract surgery. If the posterior capsule breaks during cataract surgery, vitreous gel can prolapse forward into the anterior chamber. We attempt to remove this gel via an "anterior vitrectomy" prior to putting in the new implant. The vitreous is hard to see however, as it is clear and floating in clear saline/aqueous. Kenalog can be injected into the anterior chamber: the steroid comes out as little white particles that stick to the gel surface, making it easier to visualize.

16. Eye ointments may be better than drops because:
A. less likely to wash out contacts
B. less preservative
C. quicker drug effect
D. easier to apply

The best answer is (b). Ointments tend to have less (or no) preservative because they have a very low water content. Bacteria have a difficult time growing in ointments, as they need water to thrive and replicate. This explains why peanut butter, the otherwise perfect culture medium, rarely goes bad and doesn't need refrigeration. Ointments are problematic with contact use, tend to release drug slowly, and are more difficult to use than drops.

17. Dilating drops typically have what color cap?
A. red
B. white
C. yellow
D. green

The correct answer is (a). Dilating drops usually have a red cap, while constricting drops (pilocarpine) have a green cap. The color conventions break down after this, but beta blockers like timolol often have a yellow cap.

18. After routine dilation, a 32-year-old patient complains that she can't read her phone. This is most likely secondary to what routine drop used during her exam?
A. phenylephrine
B. tropicamide
C. homatropine
D. atropine

The correct answer is (b). We typically use two eye drops to dilate patients in the clinic: phenylephrine (sympathetic stimulator) and tropicamide (short-acting parasympathetic blocker). Of these two, tropicamide has the most effect on vision as this class of drops also paralyzes the ciliary body that controls lens focus. Homatropine and atropine also have this effect but are rarely used during an adult exam as their effect lasts too long (several days). Cyclogyl (cycloplentolate) is occasionally used for refracting kids as it is strong and wears off in less than a day.

CHAPTER 4: GENERAL

19. Steroid eye drops can cause all of the following, except:
A. infection
B. glaucoma
C. delayed healing
D. iris pigmentation

The correct answer is (d). Steroid drops can increase infectious risk and is never given for patients with staining corneal ulcers or with active viral dendrites. Some patients are "steroid responders" and topical drops can make their pressure shoot up. Also, steroids are rather harsh on the ocular surface and can occasionally delay wound healing. The only drops associated with iris pigmentation are the prostaglandin drops (Xalatan, Travatan, Lumigan) that are used for glaucoma.

20. What laser is used most often by a general ophthalmologist?
A. argon
B. excimer
C. femtosecond
D. yttrium-aluminum-garnet

The correct answer is (d). The YAG laser is used primarily for removing PCO "after cataracts." We also use a variant of this YAG laser for performing SLT glaucoma treatment to the trabecular meshwork. The next most common laser is the argon, used for coagulating the iris and for treating retinal tears. The excimer and femtosecond lasers are primarily used for LASIK and other refractive surgeries. Only a small percentage of eye doctors perform refractive surgery.

21. The "A-scan" can be used for all of the following, except:
A. measuring the length of the eye
B. calculating implant power before cataract surgery
C. detecting a retinal detachment
D. grading the density of a cataract

The best answer is (d). The a-scan machine is a linear ultrasound most often used to measure the length of the eye in order to calculate implant power needed for cataract surgery. The a-scan (in combination with the b-scan) can be used to determine whether a structure floating in the vitreous cavity is a detached retina. The retina will show a dense spike on the a-scan, differentiating it from the vitreous. Cataract density can't really be graded with ultrasound.

22. A "B-scan" may be required for patients with:
A. dense cataract
B. acute glaucoma
C. wet macular degeneration
D. dendritic keratitis

The best answer is (a). A cataract can look so dense that the retina itself can't be visualized. It is useful to perform a b-scan ultrasound to make sure there are no retinal detachments or large masses behind the lens. We'd hate to perform a challenging cataract surgery on someone only to discover afterward that they had no visual potential to begin with.

23. What order should the vital signs of the eye be checked?
A. pupils, vision, pressure
B. vision, pressure, pupils
C. pressure, pupils, vision
D. vision, pupils, pressure

The correct answer is (d). We always check vision first, as penlights and numbing drops (needed for pressure measurement) can affect vision. Pupils are typically checked next since they are so easy to measure. Pressure is assessed last. I consider these three measurements to be the "vital signs" of ophthalmology, as they are measured with every patient and are essential measurements of eye function. Also, these signs need to be checked prior to dilating your patient. Remember, dilation is the time-limiting step that keeps you from going home when examining emergencies in the middle of the night.

24. Using an indirect ophthalmoscope, the image viewed is:
A. flipped
B. flipped and inverted
C. reversed

The correct answer is (b). The challenge with using the indirect ophthalmoscope is the image of the retina you see is completely backwards. Up is down and left is right. Almost all of the retina lenses we use have this issue, so you get used to it.

25. Which retinal viewing technique gives the narrowest field of view when looking at the retina?
A. direct ophthalmoscope
B. indirect ophthalmoscope
C. 90 diopter lens
D. 20 diopter lens

The best answer is (a). The direct ophthalmoscope is the little handheld device found in most non-ophthalmologists' offices. It is held very close to the eye and is meant to be used when the eye is not dilated. This gadget is very difficult to use: the retinal view you get is so small that it is very hard to get your bearings and see anything. The next narrowest view is the 90 diopter lens used at the slit-lamp for examining the posterior pole.

26. Topical numbing drops used on the eye include:
A. lidocaine
B. proparacaine
C. bupivicaine
D. marcaine

The best answer is (b). Proparacaine is the most common anesthetic eye drop we use on the eye. Tetracaine is also a common drop used in the ER, but seems to sting more going in. Lidocaine is an injectable anesthetic medicine used <u>around</u> the eye. We also use <u>preservative-free</u> lidocaine in the anterior chamber during cataract surgery. Some doctors use lidocaine jelly on the eye prior to surgery, but never in the office. Marcaine (bupivacaine) is a long-acting anesthetic not often used in ophthalmology.

27. What kind of lens is most often used at the slit-lamp to examine the retina?
A. 20 diopter
B. 28 diopter
C. 30 diopter
D. 90 diopter

The best answer is (d). The 90 diopter is a common lens used at the slit-lamp for examining the posterior pole (the central retina). It gives a great view of the macula, optic nerve, and much of the mid-periphery. The larger 20-30 diopter lenses are used during indirect ophthalmoscopy of the peripheral retina.

28. Near vision is often measured on what scale?
A. Snellen
B. Jaeger
C. Richter
D. Chromatic

The correct answer is (b). The Jaeger scale is similar to the Snellen chart, but based on "J" numbers. J1 corresponds to about 20/25 while J12 is closer to 20/100. Perfect 20/20 near-vision is often documented as J1+. Once you get worse than J3, the Jaeger scale is confusing to me, so I usually revert to Snellen equivalents when documenting near visual acuity. The Richter scale is used to measure earthquakes and the chromatic scale is used in music.

CHAPTER 4: GENERAL

29. Slit-lamp microscopes typically use:
A. white light
B. polarized light
C. black light
D. fluorescent light

The correct answer is (a). The slit-lamp microscope uses white light. Sometimes, filters (blue and green) are placed in front of the light source, but white light is the key here.

30. The swinging-light test measures:
A. absolute afferent defects
B. relative afferent defects
C. absolute efferent defects
D. relative efferent defects

The correct answer is (b). The swinging-light test is used to check the pupil response and measures the sensory (afferent) reflex. This test is only useful for measuring the light-detection of one eye relative to the other. Therefore, a defect is often described as RAPD (relative afferent pupillary defect). The other answers are made up.

31. Worldwide, the most common cause of blindness is:
A. cataract
B. glaucoma
C. diabetic retinopathy
D. trachoma

The best answer is (a). Worldwide, the most common cause of blindness is cataract. When I was a medical student, the leading cause was listed as trachoma. This is a type of Chlamydia infection spread by flies that causes chronic conjunctivitis with scarring of the inner eyelids and cornea.

CHAPTER 5
GLAUCOMA

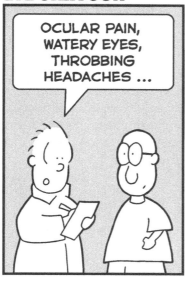
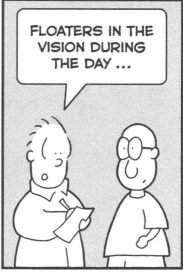
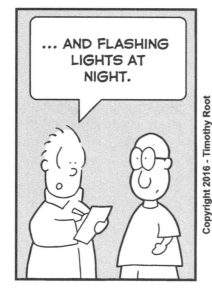
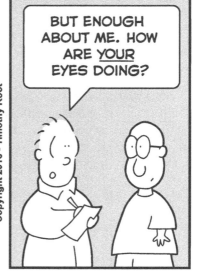

GLAUCOMA
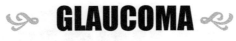
25 Questions

1. All of the following affect eye pressure measurements, except:
A. time of day
B. pupil dilation
C. thickness of cornea
D. dry eye

The best answer is (d). Many things can affect eye pressure measurements, including the time of day. This is why we document the time when we write our pressures in the chart. Corneal thickness impacts the accuracy of applanation tonometry as thicker corneas will make the pressure measurements "seem" higher than they truly are. The eye drops we use to dilate the pupil may have an effect on our measurements as well ... though this isn't a large one unless the patient goes in (or out) of angle closure. Dry eye is aggravating to the patient, but it is unrelated to eye pressure.

2. During an acute glaucoma attack, the pupil is typically:
A. miotic
B. moderately dilated
C. widely dilated
D. normal

The correct answer is (b). With acute glaucoma, the pupil is typically in a mid-dilated position and moves sluggishly (or not at all). This is because the lens has rotated forward and is shoving the iris from behind. Also, high pressure inside the eye may affect perfusion of the iris muscle and further decrease its movement.

3. Risk factors for primary glaucoma include all, <u>except</u>:
A. race
B. age
C. thin cornea
D. HLA-B27 positive

The best answer is (d). Primary glaucoma is more prevalent in black/African-Americans and in the elderly. Thin corneas have also been found to be an independent risk factor for the disease, though the underlying mechanism for this correlation is unclear. HLA-B27 disorders such as ankylosing spondylitis have been associated with uveitis (internal eye inflammation) but not directly with glaucoma.

4. Vision loss from glaucoma:
A. is permanent
B. can gradually improve
C. improves slowly with good pressure control
D. fluctuates

The best answer here is (a). Glaucoma vision loss occurs from optic nerve death. The individual ganglion nerve fibers that connect the retina to the brain atrophy and wither away. The optic nerve is part of the central nervous system, and this nerve loss is permanent. Glaucoma treatment aims to slow or stop nerve loss through lowering eye pressure. Pressure is the only glaucoma risk factor we can control.

5. Symptoms of open-angle glaucoma include:
A. floaters
B. watering
C. redness
D. nothing

The correct answer is (d). Open-angle glaucoma, often called POAG (primary open-angle glaucoma) is common and has no symptoms. Chronically elevated eye pressure gradually causes destruction of

CHAPTER 5: GLAUCOMA

the nerve fibers travelling through the optic nerve. The big problem with POAG is actually its lack of symptoms. Unless it is suspected during a screening eye exam, it may go unrecognized until vision damage becomes advanced. Floaters typically occur from breakdown of the vitreous gel inside the eye. Watering is most often caused by dry eye, and red eyes typically occur from external irritation.

6. Presenting symptoms of closed-angle glaucoma include all of the following, except:
A. halos
B. eye pain
C. peripheral vision loss
D. injection

The best answer is (c). Acute glaucoma, also called closed-angle glaucoma, is a medical emergency. The lens and iris rotate forward, blocking the flow of aqueous fluid through the pupil and closing off the drainage angle inside the eye. This causes fluid pressure to build up rapidly inside the eye, creating a ton of pain. In fact, you may find it difficult to examine your patient, as they may be busy throwing up in the trash can! Halos are very common, secondary to corneal edema. The eye will often be red from the irritation and inflammation. These patients will complain of blurry vision in general, but not peripheral vision loss. The nerve damage that occurs may eventually knock out significant amounts of their side vision, but this isn't a presenting symptom.

7. In early stages of glaucoma, people tend to loss vision in what area?
A. far peripheral vision
B. mid-peripherally
C. centrally
D. cecocentrally

The best answer is (b). While we typically tell our patients that glaucoma causes peripheral vision loss, this isn't entirely accurate. The first signs of glaucoma field loss are detected with the Humphrey visual field test as "general suppression" of their entire field. As this worsens, they start to develop localized vision loss in the mid-periphery. Their blind spot may enlarge or extend vertically in an arc pattern (an arcuate scotoma). Many people develop a "nasal step," with decreased vision medially toward the nose. Typically, the central and far peripheral vision is untouched until advanced stages. Central scotomas are more common with macular lesions (wet-macular degeneration) or direct optic nerve damage. Cecocentral scotomas occur between the central vision and blind spot and are classically associated with optic neuritis (such as with multiple sclerosis).

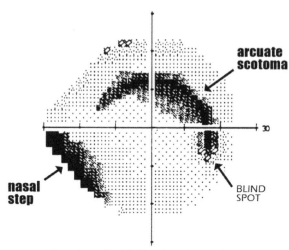

A Humphrey visual field of the right eye showing a nasal step and an arcuate defect.

8. Enlargement of the cornea from congenital glaucoma is called:
A. buphthalmos
B. exophthalmos
C. megalocornea
D. keratoglobus

CHAPTER 5: GLAUCOMA

The correct answer is (a). Buphthalmos, or "cow eye," is an enlargement of the eye (sclera and cornea) secondary to uncontrolled congenital glaucoma. The sclera and cornea are more pliable in babies and can stretch as the child matures. If you see a child with giant, beautiful eyes, rather than cooing, you should be saying to yourself "Oh, boy! Could this kid have congenital glaucoma?" Since babies don't communicate very well, the other "classic signs" of congenital glaucoma are tearing and crying (pretty nonspecific, I know). Exophthalmos is a proptosis or bulging of the eyes that is associated with thyroid disorder. Megalocornea is a rare congenital enlargement of the cornea despite normal eye pressure. Keratoglobus is a congenital thinning of the peripheral cornea that makes the entire cornea bulge out and look round or spherical. If you are a student, don't stress out over megalocornea or keratoglobus. You may never see these conditions your whole life unless you become a cornea doctor or teach at an academic ophthalmology program.

9. Acceptable laser therapy for open-angle glaucoma is:
A. ALT
B. CO2
C. LPI
D. FLT

The best answer here is (a). ALT stands for argon laser trabeculoplasty and is a laser treatment used for open-angle glaucoma. Laser spots are burned into the trabecular meshwork 360 degrees around the angle. The resulting scars improve the flow of aqueous from the eye, but also means that the procedure can't be repeated as the eye can only suffer so much scarring. ALT is being supplanted with the less aggressive SLT (selective laser trabeculoplasty) procedure that doesn't cause this scarring. The SLT procedure uses the YAG (yttrium aluminum garnet) laser, which is the same laser used during YAG capsulotomy for clearing an after-cataract opacity. LPI is a perforating laser used on the iris to break an acute glaucoma attack. FLT stands for focal laser treatment and usually describes an argon laser treatment to the retina. CO2 lasers aren't used in ophthalmology.

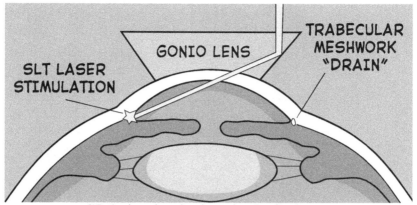

SLT stimulates the trabecular meshwork to flow better.

10. All of the following are pressure measurement techniques, except for:
A. Goldmann applanation
B. Tono-Pen applanation
C. Heidelberg tomography
D. air-puff tonometry

The correct answer is (c). Goldmann applanation is still considered the gold-standard method for checking pressure. It involves pushing (applanating) on the cornea with plastic tip illuminated with a blue light to estimate the internal pressure. The Tono-Pen is a small handheld gadget that is used to check pressure at the bedside. Air-puff tonometry is a "no touch" technique that blows air on the eye and measures the corneal reflex distortion this causes in order to estimate eye pressure. It is used more often by optometrists, and while easier to train for staff, may not be as accurate as the Goldmann. Heidelberg is not a pressure technique at all. It is a city in Germany and is sometimes used to describe the HRT (Heidelberg Retinal Tomography) used to measure the optic nerve.

CHAPTER 5: GLAUCOMA

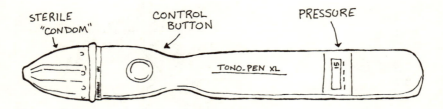

The Tono-Pen is an overpriced gadget for checking IOP at the bedside. The emergency room doesn't know how to use it and tend to get outrageous pressure readings. Competitive gadgets have come out, but the Tono-Pen is still the most common pressure machine out there for portable use.

11. What is a normal eye pressure range:
A. 5-16
B. 10-15
C. 15-32
D. 10-21

The correct answer is (d). Normal eye pressure is generally considered in the 10-21 range. Higher pressures are generally associated with glaucoma. There are many things that affect a pressure measurement, however, and "normal" is a relative term. Some people have pressure in the mid 20s and never develop glaucoma, yet others have "normal" pressure in the teens and seem to be exquisitely sensitive to mild pressure fluctuations. This is called low-tension glaucoma (LTG).

12. What prophylactic laser procedure is often performed for people at risk for acute glaucoma attacks?
A. laser peripheral iridotomy
B. laser peripheral iridectomy
C. laser peripheral iridoplasy
D. laser peripheral trabeculoplasty

The best answer is (a). Laser peripheral iridotomy (LPI) is the creation of a hole through the iris in order to equalize the pressure between the anterior and posterior chambers. In the event of pupillary block, this alternative aqueous pathway allows the iris to rotate back into its normal position, thus avoiding angle-closure attack. An iridectomy is removal of part of the iris during surgery (no lasers) and is often required when a laser can't break an attack. An iridoplasty is a shrinkage of the iris tissue using a laser. Contraction of the iris tissue keeps the peripheral iris from "bunching up" in the angle and may be needed for patients with "plateau iris." Finally, laser trabeculoplasty (ALT or SLT) is a laser applied directly to the trabecular meshwork in an attempt to lower eye pressure in people with open-angle glaucoma.

13. A blister on the conjunctiva, created during a glaucoma surgery, is called a:
A. blob
B. hot pocket
C. chemosis
D. bleb

The correct answer is (d). With trabeculectomy surgery, a drainage pathway for aqueous fluid is created that connects the anterior chamber to a pocket underneath the conjunctiva. This pocket is called a "bleb" and looks like a blister on the white of the eye. Chemosis is conjunctival swelling, often from allergies. There is no such thing as an ocular blob, and a hot pocket is a microwavable, snack famous for its colon-cleansing ability.

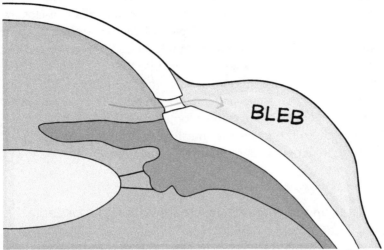

A trabeculectomy bleb filters aqueous fluid out of the anterior chamber and into the subconjunctival space to be resorbed back into the body.

14. Acute glaucoma may be treated by all of the following, except:
A. paracentesis
B. iris iridectomy
C. laser iridotomy
D. drops

The best answer is (a). A paracentesis (putting a needle in the eye) is not very effective for treating acute glaucoma. The pressure is high and there is so little room in the anterior chamber such that there is a good chance you'll run your needle through the iris and into the lens itself (creating a swollen, traumatic cataract overnight). Plus, there is little aqueous in the anterior chamber to drain, anyway. Most cases of acute glaucoma are treated with glaucoma drops (in an attempt to lower the pressure) followed by a LPI (laser peripheral iridotomy) through the iris. If this doesn't "break" the attack, the patient may need to be taken to the operating room for an surgical iridectomy (surgical creation of a hole through the iris).

15. Angles in the eye are graded on the following scale:
A. Shaffer
B. Schwalbe
C. Shaker
D. Swabee

The correct answer is (a). There are several grading systems that attempt to estimate the chance a person will have a glaucoma attack. The easiest one that we use is the Shaffer system. It is a four-point scale based on estimated corneal-iris angle seen during gonioscopy. A "Shaffer 4" means the angle is approximately 40% open, while a "Shaffer 1" is only 10% (and high risk for closing suddenly). Schwalbe's line is a very thin line seen on gonioscopy that demarcates the edge of the endothelial layer. Shakers are a Christian religious sect and swabees "clean the deck" on pirate ships.

16. Pigment dispersion syndrome is more common in:
A. hyperopes
B. myopes
C. the elderly
D. monkeys

The best answer is (b). Pigment dispersion syndrome is a type of glaucoma caused by iris pigment clogging the trabecular meshwork. The iris can bow backwards and the rub against the surface of the zonules that support the lens. The back surface of the iris is thick with pigment, which is released and then floats into the meshwork drain. This condition is more common in nearsighted people (myopes) as they have larger and deeper anterior chambers which create laxity in the iris diaphram. It also seems to be more common in young people who may have episodes of pigment release during exercise. Oddly, the condition can "burn out" and becoming less problematic with age as the enlarging lens pushes the iris forward and away from the zonules. Treatment is similar to regular glaucoma, though occasionally miotic constricting drops (like pilocarpine) are used as these tend to rotate the iris forward. An LPI can also be performed to equalize the pressure between the anterior and posterior chambers.

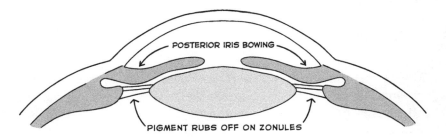

With pigment dispersion syndrome, pigment rubs off the back surface of the iris.

17. All of the following are types of glaucoma surgery hardware, except:
A. ExPress Shunt
B. Ahmed Tube Shunt
C. Baerveldt Tube
D. Malyugin Ring

The correct answer is (d). There are several glaucoma "tube shunt" devices used with advanced glaucoma, including the Molteno, Baerveldt, and Ahmed devices. These are all plastic "plates" sewn to the side of the eye, with a tube that runs into the anterior chamber. Excess fluid flows through the tube and drains into the subconjunctival space from this plate. The plate keeps the tissue from scarring down. The Mini ExPress shunt is a newer glaucoma procedure using a small metal tube. It allows the creation of a trabeculectomy bleb without as much tissue damage during surgery. The Malyugin Ring, on the other hand, is a spring-like gadget used during cataract surgery to assist with poor pupil dilation.

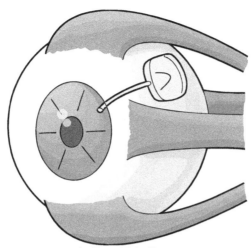

An Ahmed Tube Shunt

18. Tonometers for checking eye pressure include all of these, except:
A. Goldmann
B. Tono-Pen
C. Schiotz
D. Schulz

The correct answer is (d). The Goldmann applanation tonometer is the device bolted onto the slit-lamp microscope. It uses a blue light and pushes on the cornea to estimate internal eye pressure. The Tono-Pen is a handheld electronic device that is used at the bedside and with people who can't sit forward into the slit-lamp. The Schiotz tonometer was a really old gadget that used tiny weights to estimate eye pressure. The patient laid down flat, looking at the ceiling, as the device was pressed down onto the eye. You may never see one of these antiques in modern practice. Charles Schulz was the American cartoonist who drew Peanuts (Charlie Brown and Snoopy) and is widely considered the most influential cartoonist of all time.

CHAPTER 5: GLAUCOMA

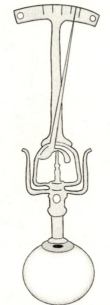

The old Schiotz tonometer

19. Pachymetry uses what technology?
A. ultrasound
B. light interference
C. oliphantine
D. reflective

The correct answer is (a). Pachymetry is the measurement of corneal thickness, and is performed using a tiny gadget that utilizes ultrasound. Corneal thickness is of prime importance in evaluating glaucoma risk and the accuracy of pressure readings. It is also of importance in patients with Fuchs' corneal dystrophy. Light interference is used with OCT, where light waves are bounced off the retina and light-wave interference patterns are compared to create a 3D view of the retinal layers (i.e. ultrasound with light). Reflective measurements are used with keratometry, a technique in which we look at the appearance of rings reflected off the tear film. Oliphant is an old derivation of elephant. It was used in the second Lord of the Rings movie, "Look Mr. Frodo, it's an oliphant!"

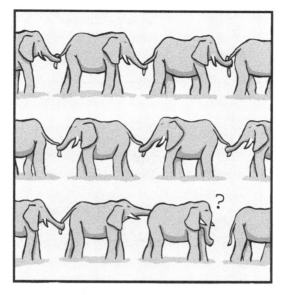

Brown-Noser
(A silly cartoon I drew years ago and never got around to publishing anywhere ... until now!)

20. Transillumination defects in the iris are seen with every condition <u>except</u>:
A. albinism
B. PXF
C. PDS
D. PDR

The correct answer is (d). Transillumination defects (TIDs) are thin areas of the iris and are usually caused by iris chaffing. We can see these defects by turning the room lights down, shooting our beam of light straight through the pupil, and seeing if any of the red-reflex shines back through the iris. This technique is useful for finding the location of prior laser LPIs and for picking up pseudoexfoliation syndrome (PXF/PEX) and pigment dispersion syndrome (PDS). Albinism can also cause transillumination through the iris from a lack of pigment. PDR (proliferative diabetic retinopathy) can cause neovascular blood vessels on the iris, but not transillumination defects.

CHAPTER 5: GLAUCOMA

21. A method for estimating anterior chamber depth is with the:
A. Van Helsing method
B. Van der Waals' method
C. Van Hagar method
D. Van Herick method

The best answer is (d). The Van Herick method is used to estimate anterior chamber depth during the slit-lamp exam. As you sweep a thin vertical of light along the cornea at 3 and 9 o'clock, you estimate the anterior chamber depth in comparison to the apparent corneal thickness. Van der Waals' force is the intermolecular forces that attract two separate molecules together. Van Hagar is the term used to describe the band Van Halen when Sammy Hagar was the lead singer. Van Helsing is the monster hunter who chases Dracula. I recommend the movie staring Hugh Jackman (it's pretty funny).

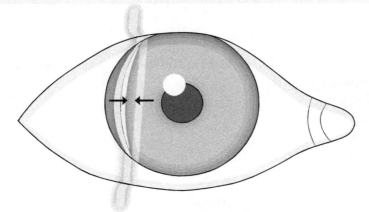

The Van Herick method for estimating anterior chamber depth.

22. Glaucoma tends to produce thinning of the optic nerve margin along what disc margins?
A. horizontal margins
B. vertical margins
C. inner margins
D. outer margins

The correct answer is (b). As the optic nerve is damaged, the cup-to-disc ratio increases, since less nerve fibers are traveling through the disc. The retina is devided into superior and inferior nerves, so we tend to see rim thinning near the inferior and superior disc margins. In fact, you might want to remember the "ISNT rule" of normal rim thickness: the inferior rim is normally thickest, followed by the superior, nasal, then temporal rims.

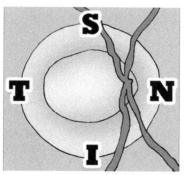 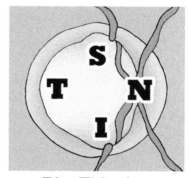

Normal Nerve **Rim Thinning**
With glaucoma, the vertical rims thin out first, breaking the ISNT rule.

23. All of the following are glaucoma drops, except:
A. timolol
B. brimonidine
C. Muro 128
D. latanoprost

The correct answer is (c). Muro 128 is a hyperosmotic salt solution used for people with cloudy corneas (usually secondary to Fuchs' dystrophy). The glaucoma drops are a little confusing to remember for the new student, so I'll list out the most common ones we use (in the class order I normally prescribe them).

1. **Prostaglandins:** Xalatan (latanoprost generic), Lumigan (bimatoprost), Travatan (travaprost)
2. **Alpha-Agonists:** Alphagan (brimonidine)
3. **Beta-Blockers:** timolol
4. **Carbonic Anhydrase Inhibitors:** dorzolamide (Trusopt), brinzolamide (Azopt)

If these don't work, we start busting out old drops like pilocarpine (also constricts the pupils) and oral Diamox (acetazolamide).

24. Potential side effects of glaucoma drops include:
A. change in iris color
B. breathing problems
C. sulfa allergy
D. paradoxical pressure elevation

The correct answer is (d). Glaucoma drops are relatively safe, though there are a few side effects you should be aware of. Prostaglandin drops like latanoprost can cause darkening of the skin around the eye, increase lash growth (women like this), and increase pigment in the iris (mostly in hazel eyes). Beta-blockers like timolol can slow the heart rate and create bronchospasm in patients with asthma or COPD. Finally, the carbonic anhydrase inhibitors (dorzolamide and oral Diamox) are sulfa-based and not good for patients with pre-existing allergy. None of the drops cause the pressure to go up, however.

25. Latanoprost is usually used at bedtime because:
A. stronger at night
B. increased half-life
C. less redness in day
D. drowsy side effects

The best answer is (c). The prostaglandin eye drops are highly effective for lowering eye pressure. However, the prostaglandin pro-inflammatory effect can make the eye red for several hours. Patients like to sleep through this redness so the eye isn't inflamed during the day.

CHAPTER 6
INFECTION

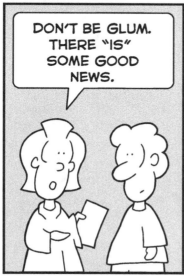
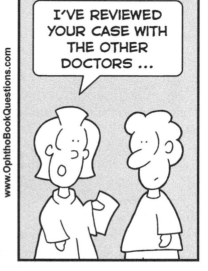
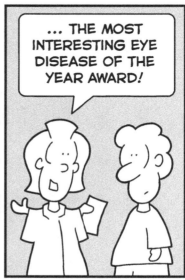

INFECTION
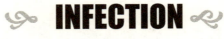
22 Questions

1. Trichoma, a common cause of blindness in the third world, is caused by:
A. protozoa
B. chlamydia
C. vitamin A deficiency
D. picornavirus

The correct answer is (b). Trichoma is a common cause of blindness is some parts of the underdeveloped world. It occurs from a type of chlamydia that infects the eyes and conjunctiva and is spread by flies. Chronic eyelid irritation causes conjunctival scarring, decreased tear production, and eventually blindness from corneal scarring. This flavor of chlamydia has a different serotype than the sexually transmitted chlamydia. The other answers are wrong, but bring up a few learning points. The protozoa we fear in the eye is toxoplasmosis (which can cause uveitis and retinal inflammation) and acanthamoeba (which causes a persistant corneal ulcer). Vitamin A deficiency can create extreme corneal drying (xerosis of the cornea) and night blindness. There aren't any high-yield diseases in the eye from picornavirus.

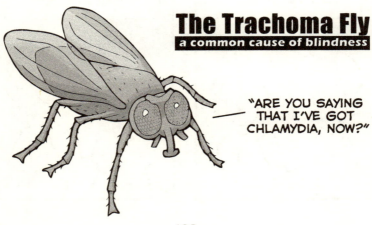

2. Herpes infection of the cornea typically presents as:
A. geographic ulcer
B. satellite lesions
C. branching pattern
D. pinpoint erosions

The best answer is (c). HSV infection of the cornea typically presents with the classic dendritic ulcer. This is a skinny, branching ulcer that looks like a branch or fern leaf. If left untreated (or if someone incorrectly treats it with topical steroids), this ulcer can enlarge into a large, geographic ulcer. Satellite lesions are a classic finding with fungal ulcers, while scattered pinpoint erosions can occur from dry eye, contact lens overwear, EKC (adenoviral infection of the cornea), or Thygeson's keratitis. Thygeson's is a poorly understood corneal inflammatory disease (and more than you need to know at the moment).

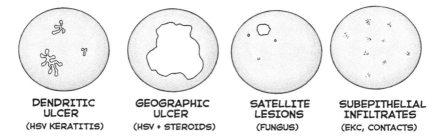

DENDRITIC ULCER (HSV KERATITIS)   GEOGRAPHIC ULCER (HSV + STEROIDS)   SATELLITE LESIONS (FUNGUS)   SUBEPITHELIAL INFILTRATES (EKC, CONTACTS)

3. An infection involving internal eye structures is a:
A. uveitis
B. endophthalmitis
C. orbitopathy
D. globe abscess

The correct answer is (b). Endophthalmitis is an infection inside the eye and universally bad. The internal eye is mostly fluid, which allows bacteria to replicate and spread rapidly, turning the interior eye into an abscess. This infection will chew up the retina and create scarring inside the eye. Treatment needs to be rapid, involving a "tap and inject" where vitreous fluid is withdrawn for culture, and antibiotics (vancomycin and ceftazidime) are injected in. The other answers are wrong. Uveitis is internal inflammation (not infection) and <u>orbitopathy</u> implies a process inside the eye socket, such as thyroid orbitopathy.

4. A hypopyon can be:
A. contagious
B. sterile
C. black
D. red

The correct answer is (b). A hypopyon is a layer of white pus in the anterior chamber. It can be a sign of internal eye infection (endophthalmitis) or sterile "reactive inflammation" from a corneal ulcer. A hypopyon is not contagious. A red layer is more likely to be blood, also known as a hyphema. I've never seen a black layer in the eye, though this could be old blood or a clot.

5. Signs of viral conjunctivitis include all, <u>except</u>:
A. papillae
B. pre-auricular node swelling
C. URI symptoms
D. pseudomembranes

The correct answer is (a). *Papillae* are small bumps on the inner eyelid, often seen with allergic conjunctivitis (and occasionally, bacterial conjunctivitis). We normally see smaller *follicles* with viral infection. In fact, the term "follicular conjunctivitis" is almost synonymous with viral infection. Viral infection often presents with a systemic prodrome, such as upper respiratory infection and signs of lymph node enlargement in front of the ear. Viral conjunctivitis can cause a ton of irritation and redness, to the point that an inflammatory "pseudomembrane" can form on the inner eyelids. These membranes are removed with forceps, as they are uncomfortable.

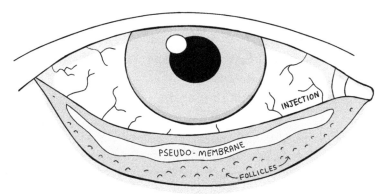

Viral conjunctivitis looks more impressive than other types of conjunctivitis.

6. What type of conjunctivitis, on average, causes the most irritation?
A. viral
B. bacterial
C. allergic
D. vernal

The best answer is (a). Viral conjunctivitis is not only the most common eye infection (at least in adults) but also tends to cause the most redness, pain, and irritation. Bacterial infection causes discharge and mucous, but not a ton of pain. Allergic and vernal (a type of seasonal allergy) conjunctivitis mainly cause itching and swelling. The periorbital swelling can be so bad with allergic conjunctivitis, that your patients may have "allergic shiners."

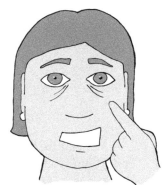

Allergic conjunctivitis can create "allergic shiners."

CHAPTER 6: INFECTION

7. Which statement best characterizes EKC infection:
A. caused by rotavirus
B. characterized by diffuse corneal edema
C. best treated with steroids
D. symptoms may last for 18 months

The best answer is (d). EKC stands for epidemic keratoconjunctivitis. It is a viral infection, like conjunctivitis, that also affects the cornea. The virus causes small, subepithelial infiltrates that can enlarge and cause larger anterior stromal scars that take many months to resolve. This condition runs as "epidemics," and is the one condition eye doctors are worried about hitting our clinic as the visual blur can knock us out for months. It is caused by a specific strain of adenovirus. There is no acute treatment for viral infections like this, though steroids may be used. This is controversial however, as steroids may actually prolong the course of the infection.

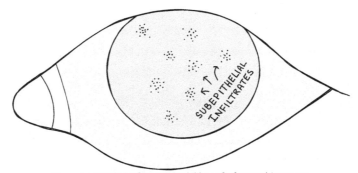

The subepithelial infiltrates look like soft, fuzzy white spots.

8. Painful infection of an eyelash follicle is best known as a:
A. hordeolum
B. chalazion
C. papillitis
D. staphyloma

The best answer is (a). The nomenclature between stye, hordeolum, and chalazion is a little confusing. A chalazion is a blockage of a large meibomian gland, deep in the eyelid. They are often nontender and sometimes necessitate draining. A stye is an infection of a lash or sweat follicle along the eyelid. The are often painful and may swell up like a pimple. A hordeolum is a general term to describe a painful inflammation of the eyelid. Whether this is an inflamed stye, chalazion, or eyelid abscess, the term hordeolum is all-encompassing and can mean *any* of them! Papillitis is a seldom-used term that describes inflammation of the optic disc. Staphyloma is a congenital eye malformation, usually involving an outpouching of the retina or optic nerve.

9. Infection of the lacrimal sac is called:
A. dacryoadenitis
B. dacryocystitis
C. dacryocystocele
D. encephalocele

The correct answer is (b). The nasolacrimal sac sits under the skin near the nose. Tears drain through this "sack" before shooting down into the nose. A blockage of the downstream passage can cause an infection to occur here. Infection in the tear drainage system can cause permanent scarring to occur, and patients may end up with epiphora (tearing) and require a drainage surgery such as a DCR. Dacryoadenitis is a rare inflammation of the lacrimal gland under the upper eyelid. Dacryocystocele is a cystic blockage in the nasolacrimal sac. This condition usually occurs in babies, and while impressive looking, this isn't an infection. Encephalocele is a downward outpouching of the brain into the orbit.

10. What oral medication is most appropriate for blepharitis?
A. doxazosin
B. doxycycline
C. diamox
D. diphenhydramine

The correct answer is (b). Oral doxycycline is sometimes prescribed for blepharitis, as it tends to improve the flow of oil throughout the body and can help with meibomian dysfunction. This antibiotic may

CHAPTER 6: INFECTION

have some anti-inflammatory properties as well, and is often used for rosacea. Doxazosin (Cardura) is an alpha-blocker that is used to relax smooth muscle and to improve urination in men suffering from BPH. Like the other "sin" medications in this class (tamsulosin and terazosin), these medications can cause floppy iris syndrome and have no role in blepharitis. Diamox is a water pill and diphenhydramine (Benadryl) is good for allergy and congestion.

11. Contact lens wearers are at particular risk for what kind of infection:
A. streptococcus
B. adenovirus
C. pseudomonas
D. moraxella

The correct answer is (c). Pseudomonas is a particularly nasty gram-negative rod that loves water. It's the bacteria that causes swimmer's ear. Contact lenses work like water sponges and tend to attract this bacteria, putting contact lens wearers at higher risk for pseudomonas ulcers. These can be particularly aggressive, and pseudomonas tends to be resistant to many antibiotics. Of the other choices, adenovirus is a common cause of viral conjunctivitis. Moraxella is associated with localized "angular blepharitis" along the outer eyelids.

12. What <u>topical</u> medication has the best pseudomonas coverage?
A. ceftazidime
B. ciprofloxacin
C. vancomycin
D. erythromycin

The correct answer is (b). Pseudomonas is a pretty nasty bacteria that's resistant to many antibiotics. The topical antibiotics I use the most for pseudomonas are the fluoroquinolones (ciprofloxacin, gatifloxacin, moxifloxacin, and besifloxacin) and tobramycin. Fortified vancomycin is great for gram-positive infections and

MRSA, but almost all pseudomonas are resistant to it. Erythromycin is a great antibiotic for prophylactic infection coverage (such as after a non-dirty corneal abrasion), but the ointment isn't strong enough for an active ulcer infection. Ceftazidime has wonderful pseudomonas activity, but it not available topically - instead, it is injected inside the eye (along with vancomycin) during a tap-and-inject for endophthalmitis. I know this is confusing, so here is the breakdown of my personal antibiotic preferences:

CONJUNCTIVITIS OR SMALL, CLEAN CORNEAL ABRASION
erythromycin ointment
DIRTY ABRASION OR A CONTACT LENS WEARER
ciprofloxacin
SMALL CORNEAL ULCER
double cover with gatifloxacin/besifloxacin and tobramycin
LARGE CORNEAL ULCER
fortified vancomycin and fortified tobramycin
ENDOPHTHALMITIS
tap-and-inject with vancomycin and ceftazidime

13. Signs of orbital cellulitis include all, except:
A. enophthalmos
B. chemosis
C. diplopia
D. APD

The correct answer is (a). Orbital cellulitis causes inflammation behind the eye. This can involve the eye muscles and cause diplopia, as well as optic nerve dysfunction causing an APD. Chemosis is a swelling of the conjunctiva and a non-specific sign of inflammation of the eye. Inflammation behind the eye will make the eye bulge outwards (proptosis). Enophthalmos is a *retraction* of the globe and usually occurs after traumatic fracture of the sinus bones. Another (extremely rare) cause of enophthalmos is metastatic breast cancer that can cause fibrosis of the intraorbital contents with resulting contracture of the eyeball.

CHAPTER 6: INFECTION

14. Dendritic corneal ulcers are most associated with:
A. herpes zoster
B. herpes simplex 1
C. herpes simplex 2
D. varicella zoster

The correct answer is (b). Most herpetic eye disease is caused by HSV1. This is the same virus rampant in the general population that causes cold sores (i.e. not an STD, like HSV2). These dendritic ulcers form on the corneal surface, with a classic appearance that is easily diagnosed when stained with fluorescein. Varicella zoster (chicken pox and shingles) is the virus that causes herpes zoster of the eye ... the corneal lesions zoster cause are called "pseudodendrites" and look raised with an inverse fluorescein staining along their edges.

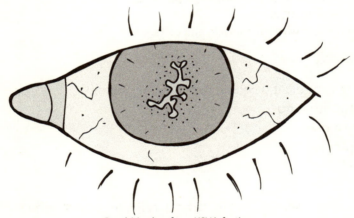

Dendritic ulcer from HSV infection

15. Initial treatment for a dendritic corneal ulcer may include all, <u>except</u>:
A. trifluridine
B. ganciclovir
C. Tobradex
D. acyclovir

The correct answer is (c). HSV infections require antiviral treatment. The mainstay in the USA is still topical trifluridine (more commonly called Viroptic). This antiviral drop works well, but must be dosed fairly often (5-9 times a day) and is very harsh on the cornea. Ganciclovir is now available as a topical ointment (Zirgan) that is better tolerated, though expensive. Topical acyclovir hasn't been FDA approved in the USA for eye use, and it probably never will: the agent is not profitable enough for a drug company to bother. Oral antivirals, like acyclovir or valacyclovir, are often used in conjunction with topical treatment. You wouldn't use an antibiotic/steroid drop like Tobradex (tobramycin/dexamethasone) with a dendritic cornea - the steroid can make the dendrites grow and grow, becoming a massive geographic ulcer. In general, steroids are dangerous to use with any corneal abrasion or ulcer, as they can help bacteria/virus/fungus grow faster.

16. Most types of adult conjunctivitis are:
A. bacterial
B. viral
C. allergic
D. psychosomatic

The correct answer is (b). Most cases of conjunctivitis are viral, often caused by adenovirus in association with cold or flu symptoms. This is true in adults, but in young children bacteria may be more likely. When kids have conjunctivitis, I tend to always treat them with a mild, well-tolerated antibiotic like erythromycin ointment.

17. Eyelid follicles are associated with:
A. bacterial infection
B. viral infection
C. allergic reaction
D. chemical reaction

The best answer is (b). Follicles are small red bumps seen on the inner eyelids (the palpebral conjunctiva). They are associated with viral infection. Larger papillae bumps are seen with allergic reactions, especially with GPC (giant papillary conjunctivitis), a kind of allergic reaction to contact lens overwear. Bacteria also tend to cause larger papillae. None of these findings are very specific, unfortunately.

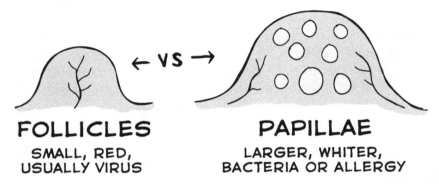

Follicles and papillae are common, but not as diagnostically useful as you might think.

18. Homemade saline solution has been associated with:
A. methanol blindness
B. protozoa infection
C. hyponatremia
D. corneal edema

The correct answer is (b). Apparently, back in the 70s and early 80s, it was popular for contact lens wearers to make their own homemade saline solution. This drastically increased people's risk for protozoa infection with acanthamoeba. This nasty water-borne germ is found throughout nature and often in tap water (especially in the UK and places with roof-top water towers). It causes a terrible, painful corneal ulcer. The diagnosis of acanthamoeba is difficult (corneal scrapings) and the treatment is tricky (topical "pool cleaners"). The infection is difficult to diagnose without getting a corneal sample, and many of these people require a corneal transplant.

19. Where does a keratitis infection occur?
A. conjunctiva
B. sclera
C. carrots
D. cornea

The correct answer is (d). The prefix kerato- is used to describe the cornea: example keratoplasty (transplant), keratoconus (cone-shaped cornea), and keratoprosthesis (prosthetic eye). A keratitis is an infection or inflammation of the cornea. This is fairly uncommon, and often secondary to virus. Examples of this might be herpetic HSV keratitis or EKC (epidemic keratoconjunctivitis from adenovirus). A keratitis can cause corneal scarring, so it is more dangerous than a conjunctivitis.

20. Giant papillary conjunctivitis occurs most frequently in:
A. school-aged children
B. contact lens wearers
C. prostitutes
D. zombies

The correct answer is (b). GPC is usually caused by contact lens overwear and looks like giant papillae bumps on the inside of the upper eyelid. The pathogenesis is a little unclear, but this condition is likely a reaction to irritants within the contact lens. Most patients complain that they can't keep their contact in their eye for long without the eye becoming irritated. Treatment involves artificial tears, mild steroids, and a contact lens holiday.

CHAPTER 6: INFECTION

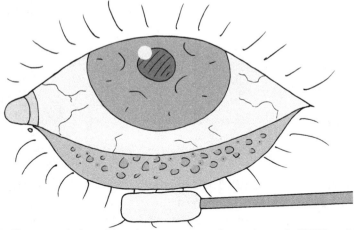

GPC bumps on the inner lids ... they are even more impressive on the UPPER eyelid!

21. Appropriate coverage for a large corneal ulcer is:
A. erythromycin and ceftriaxone
B. ciprofloxacin
C. fortified ofloxacin and Tobradex
D. fortified vancomycin and tobramycin

The best answer is (d). When we have a large corneal ulcer, it is usually best to use the "big guns" for antibiotic coverage. This usually means using vancomycin (MRSA coverage) and tobramycin (to cover pseudomonas). Vancomycin isn't normally available as an eye drop, so both these medications can be mixed up by a compounding pharmacy as high strength "fortified" antibiotics. As far as the other choices, erythromycin ointment isn't appropriate as too many bacteria are resistant and it's not terribly "strong." Fluoroquinolones like ciprofloxacin can be a good choice (especially in contact lens wearers), but the fourth generation medicines like gatifloxacin or besifloxacin may have better overall single-agent coverage. Remember, it's safest to use two antibiotics when you have a large, vision-threatening ulcer! Tobradex contains steroids - steroids are a big no-no when treating ulcers since they'll suppress the immune response and allow the bacteria to flourish. Ceftriaxone is given via IV in a hospital setting. We only use IV ceftriaxone with ocular gonorrhea, which produces so much watering and nasty mucous discharge that topical antibiotics wash out too quickly.

22. A patient complains of a "yellow bump" on the white of their eye. This is most likely a:
A. papilloma
B. pterygium
C. pinguecula
D. pseudomonas

The best answer is (c). A pinguecula is a thickened area of conjunctival skin that occurs on the white of the eye. These occur from chronic wind and sun exposure and are more common in outdoor professions like construction and beach lifeguards. When a pinguecula enlarges, it can grow over the surface of the cornea. This is called a pterygium. Papilloma is a general term used to describe skin tags that occur around the eye, usually along the eyelid margin. Pseudomonas is a bacteria common in water and soil that can cause a nasty corneal infection, especially common in contact lens wearers.

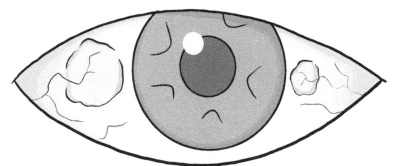

Pinguecula ... same mechanism as a pterygium but doesn't extend over the cornea.

CHAPTER 7
LIDS&LACRIMATION

EYE CARTOON   by Tim Root, M.D.

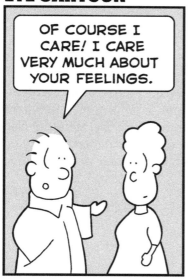
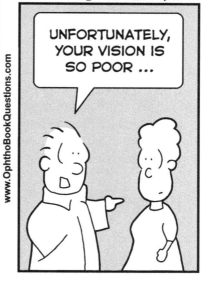
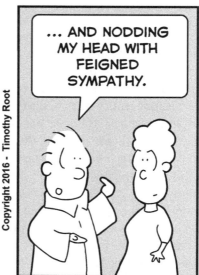

LIDS & LACRIMATION

22 Questions

1. Dry eye may be exacerbated by all, <u>except</u>:
A. age
B. thyroidopathy
C. rheumatoid arthritis
D. cataract surgery

The best answer is (d). Dry eye is fairly common as we get older. Also, thyroid disease can dry the eye and cause exposure dryness from lid retraction. Rheumatoid arthritis and other autoimmune diseases can cause Sjogren's syndrome, where the excretory glands producing tears and saliva are destroyed. Cataract surgery may cause short-term irritation, but doesn't exacerbate dry eye.

2. A test for dry eye is:
A. Schirmer's test
B. Schilling test
C. Turing test
D. dye disappearance test

The correct answer is (a). The Schirmer's test involves placing a small piece of filter paper over the eyelid margin and measuring the amount of tears produced along the filter. I've never found it particularly useful in daily practice, but some purists still do it. The dye disappearance test is performed by placing fluorescein in the eye and seeing if this dye disappears over time. If it doesn't, this may indicate a blockage of the nasolacrimal system. The Schilling test isn't performed by eye doctors, but is used for measuring B12 absorption in cases of pernicious anemia. The Turing test was proposed by Alan Turing, and was intended to be used as a method for measuring artificial intelligence. If a person could have a conversation with a computer and an impartial judge couldn't tell if a machine was involved, that machine "intelligence" was said to have passed the Turing test. Alan Turing was an important pioneer in computing and code breaking during World War 2. Unfortunately, his life was ignominiously cut short after a tragic incident involving a young man, forced chemical castration, and a poisoned apple. Look it up.

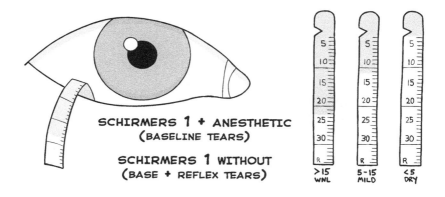

3. The surface layer of the tear film is made of:
A. aqueous
B. mucous
C. oil
D. vinegar

The correct answer is (c). The tear film is formed from three layers. The bottom most layer is the mucous layer that helps the tears spread and stick to the eye. The aqueous is the middle watery component of the tears. The surface layer is a layer of oil lipid. This oil layer is produced by the meibomian glands, and is important for surface tension and for creating an evaporation barrier to keep the tears from dissipating too quickly.

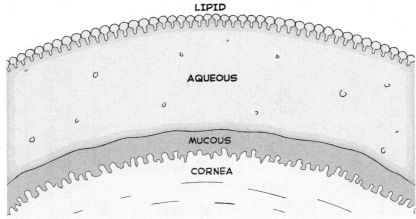
The three layers of the tear film - lipid, aqueous, and mucous

4. A patient complains that her dry eyes have gotten worse, despite increasing the frequency of her artificial tears. She may be suffering from:
A. medicamentosa
B. fibromyalgia
C. toxic drop syndrome
D. the "sugar"

The best answer is (a). Medicamentosa is when a medication, such as eye drops, causes more harm than it is helping (usually from overuse). Artificial tears contains preservatives that can irritate the cornea epithelium when used too frequently. Fibromyalgia is a sensory condition where people have multiple complaints in different systems (including dry eye and chronic eye irritation). Toxic drop syndrome (TDS) is completely made up but sounds legitimate, right? The "sugar" is a fun way to say diabetes.

5. An inward turning of the eyelid is called:
A. entropion
B. ectropion
C. trichiasis
D. introversion

The correct answer is (a). Entropion is an inward turning of the eyelid, often resulting in the lashes rubbing against the eye. Like ectropion (outward turning of the lid), this usually occurs due to laxity of the lid layers from aging. Trichiasis is an inward turning of the eyelashes. Introversion means that you are shy and fear social interaction.

6. A blepharoplasty is done to treat:
A. blepharitis
B. dermatochalsis
C. conjunctivochalasis
D. blepharosaurus

The best answer is (b). A blepharoplasty is the surgical removal of excess skin of the eyelid ... also known as dermatochalasis. Blepharitis is inflammation of the eyelids that causes chronic eye irritation. Conjunctivochalasis is stretching of the conjunctival skin so that it sags and becomes irritated with blinking. The blepharosaurus is a mythical dinosaur, known for his long neck and chronic ocular irritation.

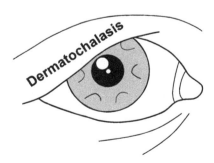

7. Basal tears are produced by which of the following gland(s)?
A. lacrimal
B. Krause and Wolfring
C. nasolacrimal
D. Walsh and Hoyt

The correct answer is (b). Basal tears are actually produced by the glands of Krause and Wolfring. These glands are similar to the larger lacrimal gland, but smaller, more numerous, and located on the inner surface of the lids way up under the eyelid in the fornix. The lacrimal gland is only responsible for reflex tearing. There is no such thing as the nasolacrimal gland. Walsh and Hoyt wrote a big, famous book on neuro-ophthalmology.

8. When tears leave the eye, what is the correct order of passage:
A. puncta, canaliculi, sac, nasolacrimal duct
B. puncta, sac, canaliculi, nasolacrimal duct
C. puncta, sac, nasolacrimal duct, canaliculai
D. canaliculi, puncta, sac, nasolacrimal duct

The correct answer is (a). Tears drain from the eye into the nose via the nasolacrimal system. This includes the punctum "holes" located on the surface of the inner eyelids. Tears then drain through small canalicular ducts into the lacrimal sac. From here, tears drain down through the thin nasolacrimal duct into the nose.

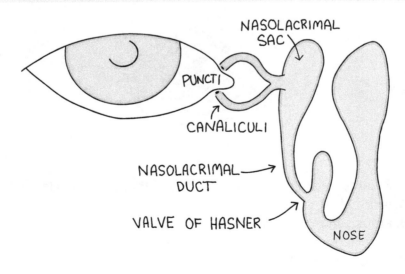

9. If a person has a complete blockage of the nasolacrimal duct, what surgery will be required?
A. NLD probing
B. DCR
C. Jones tube
D. septoplasty

The correct answer is (b). Infection in the nasolacrimal system causes inflammation and scarring within the nasolacrimal duct. This leads to chronic tearing and mucous buildup, as tears can no longer drain into the nose. Treatment usually requires a DCR (dacryocystorhinostomy) with an oculoplastics or ENT specialist. This involves making an external skin incision to enter the nasolacrimal sac. A hole is then punched from the sac directly into the nasal cavity. This bypasses the nasolacrimal duct entirely. Probing may help with duct obstruction in children, as they usually have an imporforate Valve of Hasner (where the duct drains into the nose). However, probing is unlikely to be effective in adults with complete duct blockage. A septoplasty is for correcting a deviated septum in the nose.

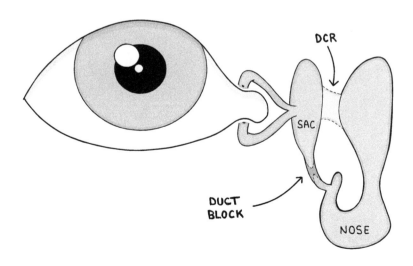

10. If a person has a blockage of both upper and lower canaliculi, what surgery may be required?
A. punctoplasty
B. cannalectomy
C. Jones tube
D. DCR

The best answer is (c). If the canaliculi are blocked, then tears can't reach the rest of the nasolacrimal sac and duct, making the whole system useless. In this case, a Jones tube is required. A direct pathway from the medial eyelid into the nose is created, and a skinny glass tube is placed to allow the tears to flow through. A punctoplasty is a snip procedure performed on the punctum in an attempt to widen the hole. I've never heard of a cannalectomy. A DCR is performed for nasolacrimal duct obstruction and involves breaking through the bone at the nasolacrimal sac.

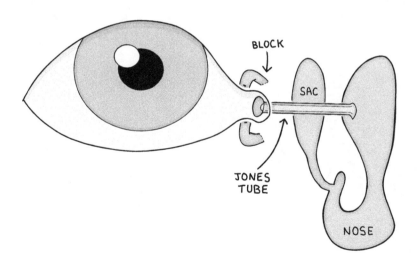

11. A Crawford tube might be used for all, except:
A. nasolacrimal stenosis
B. traumatic cannalicular damage
C. dacryoadenitis
D. imperforate valve of Hassner

The best answer is (c). A Crawford tube is a small silicone tube with the thickness of angel-hair pasta. It is often threaded through the nasolacrimal system in order to keep the pathway patent after surgeries. For example, if a patient has a traumatic eyelid injury, their canaliculus pathway may be cut. When possible, a Crawford tube is threaded through the severed canaliculus, and the wound is repaired around the tube. Several months later, the Crawford tube can be removed and, hopefully, the canalicular pathway will remain intact. The tube is sometimes placed in children with NLD (nasolacrimal duct) obstruction. This is usually secondary to an imperforate valve of Hasner within the nose. Dacryoadenitis is an inflammation of the lacrimal gland in the upper eyelid and unrelated to the nasolacrimal drainage system.

12. The epicanthal fold is:
A. seen *only* with Down syndrome
B. prominent in youth
C. absent in Asians
D. formed by the levator insertion

The best answer is (b). An epicanthal fold is a fold of tissue seen nasally, common in Asians, children, and people with Down syndrome. The levator inserts onto the eyelid tarsus to create the upper lid crease. A prominent epicanthal fold can cause pseudoesotropia - the illusion of crossed eyes.

13. The tarsus is a:
A. suspensory ligament
B. plate of connective tissue
C. canthal insertion
D. periosteal rim

The correct answer here is (b). The tarsal plate is a tough tissue deep within the eyelids that gives the lids their firmness and integrity. The tarsal plate has the consistency of cartilage, like that found in our ears, but it is NOT actually made of cartilage. The tarsal plate is much larger in our upper eyelid, and serves as an attachment point for the levator muscle to pull the eyelid up. The meibomian glands are also embedded within the tarsus. The other answers are incorrect. While there ARE suspensory ligaments within the orbit that hold the eye in place (like a sling or hammock), these ligaments are confusing, have little clinical relevance, and are quite beyond the scope of a beginning student. The canthus is the insertion point of the eyelids. We have both a lateral canthus and a medial canthus (near the nose). The periosteal rim is the tissue running on the surface of bone. If someone has a loose or lax eyelid, the eyelid can be detached from the lateral canthus and resewn to the periosteum deeper inside the orbital rim. This procedure is called a lateral tarsal strip and a common treatment for ectropion (outward lid rotation).

14. A chalazion is drained by making an incision through:
A. external eyelid
B. palpebral conjunctiva
C. lid margin
D. canthus

The correct answer is (b). A chalazion occurs after blockage of a meibomian gland. These glands sit deep in the eyelid, embedded in the tarsal plate. To drain a chalazion, the eyelid is flipped over and a scalpel is used through the palpebral conjunctiva and into the tarsal plate. This incision is made vertically to avoid damaging neighboring meibomian glands. We try to avoid draining through the external eyelid to avoid scarring, though this is occasionally done if the chalazion is right under the surface. You never make incisions at the lid margin as this might create a notch in the eyelid contour. The canthus is the corner of the eyelid where the upper and lower lids connect.

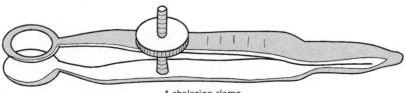

A chalazion clamp

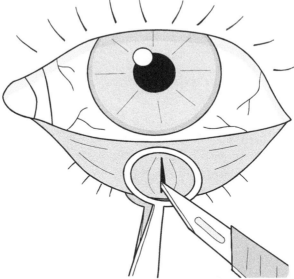
Chalazions are incised and drained from the inside of the eyelid.

15. A good testing device for bulging eyes is the:
A. Hertel exophthalmometer
B. Riddick exophthalmometer
C. Avery exophthalmometer
D. Goldmann exophthalmometer

The correct answer is (a). The Hertel exophthalmometer (good luck with the pronunciation) is a ruler held up to the eyes to measure how far the eyes protrude in relation to the lateral orbital rim. When we say "Goldmann," we are usually talking about Goldmann applanation (pressure checking) or the old Goldmann visual field test machine. Riddick is a science fiction movie character with odd glowing eyes, played by Vin Diesel. There are no devices invented by Riddick, but there is a weird neurology disorder called the Riddoch syndrome where people can only see moving objects (not high yield). Tex Avery is a cartoonist and animator with Warner Brothers who invented Bugs Bunny and Daffy Duck.

CHAPTER 7: LIDS & LACRIMATION

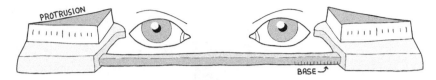

The Hertel is simply a ruler with mirrors used for measuring eye protrusion.

16. Thyroid orbitopathy may show all of the following, <u>except</u>:
A. enlargement of the rectus muscle belly
B. enlargement of tendon insertions
C. lid retraction
D. exophthalmos

The correct answer is (b). Thyroid orbitopathy (Graves' disease) causes proptosis (exophthalmos) of the globe and occurs secondary to swelling of the intraorbital muscles and fat-pads. On CT scan, the eye muscles have classic enlargement of the muscle bellies with sparing of the tendon insertions on the eye. This is in contrast to orbital inflammation (pseudotumor of the orbit), which causes enlargement of everything (tendons and all). Thyroid dysfunction is the main cause of upper-lid retraction as well.

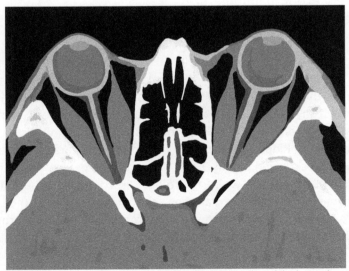

With thyroid disease, the rectus muscle belly looks swollen while the tendon insertion on the eyeball is still skinny.

17. Chalazions have all the following features, <u>except</u>:
A. they occur in meibomian glands
B. they tend to be painless
C. they are filled with keratin
D. they are associated with pyogenic granuloma

The best answer is (c). A chalazion occurs when one of the deep, oil-producing meibomian glands clogs up. This leads to the formation of a large, usually painless bump in the eyelid that may need to be drained if it doesn't resolve. Chalazions are filled with white, <u>oily</u> pus and are often associated with pyogenic granulomas. A pyogenic granuloma is an inflammatory red bump that forms on the inner eyelid. They often melt away with steroid drops, but may need to be excised if they become large or recalcitrant. Keratin is a white, waxy substance - there <u>are</u> lesions on the eyelids that contain keratin, such as the harmless keratin-filled inclusion cyst.

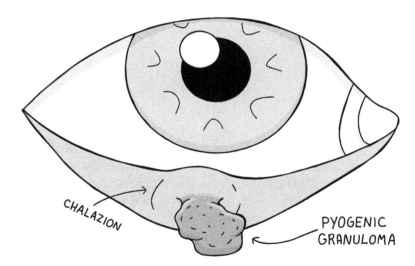

A pyogenic granuloma can form next to a chalazion. They will often melt away with topical steroids. Larger ones may need excision.

CHAPTER 7: LIDS & LACRIMATION

18. Exam findings consistent with blepharitis include all, except:
A. telangiectasia of eyelid margin
B. lash collarettes
C. punctuate epithelial erosions
D. frothy tears

The best answer is (c). Blepharitis is chronic irritation of the eyelids. Patients can have dilated telangiectatic vessels on their lids, especially people with co-existing rosacea. Anterior blepharitis may cause collarettes of debris to form around the base of eyelashes and posterior blepharitis may affect meibomian oil secretions and make the tears look frothy with little bubbles along the lid margin. Punctate epithelial erosions (PEEs) are small spots of staining found on the cornea, and are usually a sign of dry eye.

19. A chalazion can cause all, except:
A. tumor
B. amblyopia
C. astigmatism
D. ptosis

The correct answer is (a). A chalazion is a swelling of a meibomian gland that causes a painless bump in the eyelid. Normally, this bump is unsightly but inconsequential. If large enough, the chalazion can cause the eyelid to droop (ptosis) and push on the eye itself, causing some astigmatism blur. This is a big deal in an infant: any lid droop can cause amblyopia, and chalazion are therefore monitored closely in babies. A chalazion can't CAUSE a tumor, though a rare sebaceous tumor of the eyelid can masquerade as a recurrent chalazion.

20. Lid retraction can be caused by all of the following, except:
A. dilating drops
B. thyroid
C. contralateral ptosis
D. Horner's syndrome

The best answer is (d). Horner's syndrome is a loss of sympathetic tone to the eye. It causes a mild ptosis (droopy eyelid) from loss of innervation to Mueller's muscle in the upper eyelid. The other answers listed all cause the eyelid to retract. Phenylephrine dilating drops stimulate the iris retractors *and* Mueller's muscle to lift the lid. Thyroid dysfunction is a common cause for lid retraction. Another cause is droopiness in the *other* eye - in an attempt to raise the droopy lid, the normal eye will raise too high.

21. Trichiasis is when the eyelashes:
A. grow in toward the eye
B. come out of the meibomian gland orifices
C. stop growing from chronic inflammation
D. lose their pigmentation and look white

The best answer is (a). Trichiasis is when the eyelashs grow in the wrong direction, pointing inward towards the eye. Distichiasis is when lashes grow out of the meibomian orifices. Madarosis is a loss of lash growth, often from chronic blepharitis. Poliosis is a loss of pigmentation in the lashes.

22. Superior limbic keratoconjunctivitis is related to:
A. rheumatoid arthritis
B. ankylosing spondylitis
C. thyroid disorder
D. dry eye

The best answer is (c). SLK is a combination of keratitis (irritation of the cornea) and conjunctivitis that seems to target the conjunctiva under the upper eyelid. This is a strange location for ocular irritation, as the superior conjunctiva is usually covered by the upper eyelid and well lubricated. This condition occurs more often with thyroid disorder - this makes sense, because these patients tend to have dry eye and upper lid retraction (though this probably isn't the underlying mechanism of SLK). These patients complain of chronic ocular irritation and tend to switch doctors because no one can find anything wrong. They will exhibit staining of the conjunctival surface with rose bengal (or lissamine green) dye and have large bumps under their eyelid that looks like contact lens GPC. Treatment is challenging. In the past, silver nitrate cauterization of the conjunctiva and conjunctival resection have been tried. Most eye doctors begin conservatively with lubrication, punctal plugs, and large diameter contact lenses.

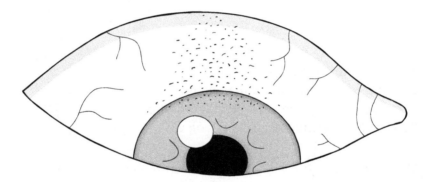

SLK is associated with thyroid dysfunction

CHAPTER 8
NEURO

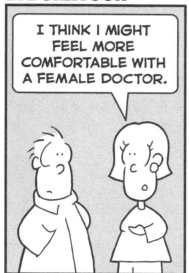
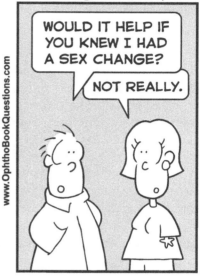
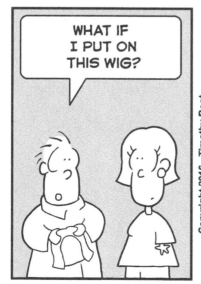
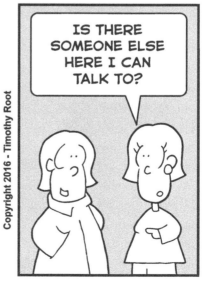

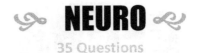

NEURO
35 Questions

1. Confrontational fields can be measured using:
A. fingers
B. Humphrey
C. Goldmann
D. all of the above

The correct answer is (d). Peripheral vision can be measured several ways. Most patients are simply checked by finger counting. The Humphrey visual field machine is used for patients with glaucoma or stroke. It works by shining a spot of light on the inside of a white bowl. Whenever patients see the spot in their peripheral vision, they click a buzzer and the Humphrey computer subsequently maps out their vision. The Goldmann field is an older manual technique that involves a larger bowl of light and a moving light target. Patient responses are manually drawn on grid paper. Goldmann fields are time-consuming, and usually reserved for patients with extremely bad vision that can't be mapped with a HVF (Humphrey visual field). Few people enjoy administering the Goldmann field as the test requires constant supervision and coaching. The Goldmann machine is no longer built - this test is slowly phasing out as the machines break down.

2. When describing the eye movements, it is important to comment on:
A. ductions and versions
B. intorsions and extorsions
C. speed and smooth pursuit
D. feng and shui

The best answer is (a). Ductions are how each eye moves independently. In other words, an eye can abduct, adduct, etc. Versions, on the other hand, describe how the eyes move together - such as convergence inwards, or divergence outwards. Incyclotorsions and extorsions are important, certainly, but difficult to measure and rarely a problem except in 4th nerve palsies and higher level problems like congenital DVD (dissociated vertical deviation) and myokymias - too high a level to worry about here. Eye movement speed and smooth pursuit is only important with certain types of brain lesions and intoxication. Finally, feng shui is only important to bad interior designers.

3. Horner's syndrome is associated with:
A. pupillary dilation
B. increased perspiration
C. ptosis
D. RAPD

The best answer is (c). Horner's syndrome occurs with damage to the sympathetic input to the eye. The sympathetic system (our "fight or flight" system) makes the pupil dilate, increases perspiration, and lifts our eyelid (presumably, so we can see better as we run away from attacking bears in the middle of the night). If this pathway is damaged, the opposite occurs. Our pupil constricts, we get anhydrosis (decreased sweating), and the eyelid droops a little. Horner's will not cause an APD, however, as the optic nerve is not damaged so there is no sensory deficit.

CHAPTER 8: NEURO

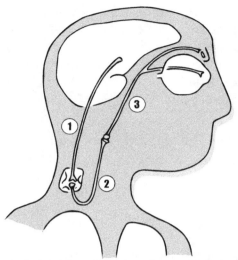

The sympathetic chain is long. Horner's syndrome can indicate a problem anywhere along this path, including the neck and lung apex.

4. Asymmetric pupils are:
A. anisochromic
B. anisometric
C. anisocoric
D. aniseikonic

The correct answer is (c). Anisocoria is when the pupils are of different sizes. Anisochromia is when the eyes are of different color, though this is usually described as heterochromia. Anisometropia is when the prescription between the eyes is very different, which makes it difficult for people to adjust to their glasses. Aniseikonia is when there is a difference in the perceived size of objects between the two eyes. For example, if a patient has macular edema in one eye, their photoreceptors will be spread out, making objects appear smaller in that eye. If you found this nomenclature confusing, you may be suffering from anisocomprendia (yes, I made that up - I'll stop now).

5. A dilated pupil is considered to be:
A. miotic
B. mydriatic
C. adriatic
D. instamatic

The correct answer is (b). A dilated pupil is said to have mydriasis and "mydriatic drops" are used to intentionally dilate the pupil. In contrast, miotic drops such as pilocarpine make the pupils constrict, becoming smaller. The Adriatic is the sea next to Italy. The Instamatic was a series of inexpensive, easy-to-load film cameras made by Kodak in 1963 that helped usher in low-cost photography to the masses.

6. Pupils will constrict with all, <u>except</u>:
A. accommodation
B. refixation
C. pilocarpine
D. inflammation

The correct answer is (b). Pupils constrict with light (obviously) but they also constrict when focusing on near objects (accommodation). This constriction helps with focusing as small pupil aperture improves depth of focus. Pilocarpine is a miotic drop used to constrict the pupils. Internal ocular inflammation (iritis/uveitis) often causes the pupil to constrict as well. Refixation and "just looking around" doesn't affect the pupil size, unless you refixate and look at the sun (or at something close up).

7. What will make the pupils dilate?
A. looking at food
B. a first kiss
C. eating popcorn
D. smelling black licorice

CHAPTER 8: NEURO

The best answer is (b). Pupillary dilation is controlled by the sympathetic fight-flight system. Stressful situations like a first kiss or meeting a horny bear in the woods causes this reflex to kick in. Your pupils dilate so that you can see better in the dark as you run away. Conversely, the parasympathetic rest-digest reflex causes the pupil to constrict when eating and when focusing on near objects like food.

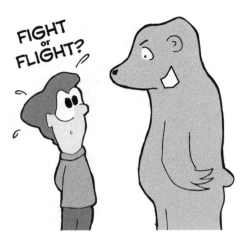

"Pucker up little fella!"

8. If you have a right sixth nerve palsy, what direction would you turn your head to avoid double vision?
A. right
B. left
C. up
D. down

The correct answer is (a). If you had a right sixth nerve palsy, you would have crossed eyes with your right eye turned in toward your nose. To see straight ahead without double vision, you would have to turn your head to the right to get both eyes in alignment.

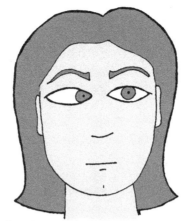

Diplopic patients may have to turn their heads to get both eyes looking in the same direction.

9. A cover-uncover test is best at detecting:
A. tropia
B. phoria
C. version
D. duction

The correct answer is (a). A tropia is a misalignment between the eyes such as esotropia (cross-eyed) and exotropia (wall-eyed). If the alignment issue is large, diagnosis is easy. Many times, however, the alignment problem is small. In these cases we can perform the cover-uncover test. While having your patient stare at a fixed point, you cover, then uncover each eye. If you see a refixation movement when an eye is uncovered, then you know the eye was out of alignment.

10. Cross-cover testing detects:
A. tropia
B. phoria
C. tropia plus phoria
D. tropia minus phoria

CHAPTER 8: NEURO

The correct answer is (c). Ocular alignment problems are usually broken down into phorias and tropias. A tropia is an alignment problem that is always present (such as cross-eyed esotropia) and is picked up using the cover-uncover test. A phoria, however, is an alignment problem that is only discovered when fusion between the eyes is broken. This can be elicited by covering each eye, back and forth, never letting the eyes fixate at the same time. This keeps the eyes from working together and a phoric eye may wander out of alignment. This form of cross-cover testing is primarily used for measuring phorias, but <u>technically</u> the test measures their phoria, <u>plus</u> any full-time tropia. Don't worry if this seems confusing; you may want to watch my lecture on "Tropia versus Phoria" at OphthoBook.com (or YouTube) to learn more about cover testing.

11. Pupil abnormalities are usually detected using the:
A. cover-uncover test
B. cross-cover test
C. swinging light test
D. lantern test

The correct answer is (c). The swinging light test is the main (and only) test we use for checking the pupils. It involves swinging a bright light back and forth between the pupils, making sure that the pupils constrict with each pass. If the pupils dilate when the light hits one eye, there is a pupil defect. The cover-uncover test is used for checking tropias and the cross-cover test for phorias. I've never performed a "lantern test" - I made the term up, though there is a Farnsworth lantern test used for detecting color-blindness in aviator pilots.

12. An Adie's tonic pupil is often caused by:
A. quinine toxicity
B. viral infection
C. endophthalmitis
D. vacuum decompression

The correct answer is (b). Adie's pupil is a dilated pupil that occurs from damage to the ciliary ganglion located behind the eyeball within the eye socket. This damage often occurs after a harmless viral infection and is more common in young woman (average age around 30). They present to the office after friends point out their pupils are the wrong size. Endophthalmitis is an internal ocular infection that usually occurs after surgery. Quinine is an ancient medicine derived from the cinchona tree that has anti-inflammatory properties and was the first treatment for malaria. It can be toxic in high quantities, but rarely used except in minute quantities in tonic water (i.e. gin and tonic drinks). Vacuum decompression happens to astronauts.

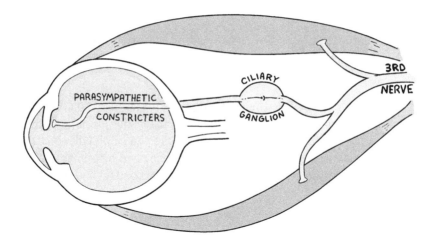

The parasympathetic "constrictor" nerves run with the third cranial nerve and pass through the ciliary ganglion before innervating the iris. An Adie's pupil occurs from damage at the ganglion and creates a dilated pupil (but no double vision).

13. An Adie's Pupil is:
A. dilated at distance but constricts at near
B. dilated at distance and near
C. constricted at distance and dilates at near
D. constricts at distance and near

CHAPTER 8: NEURO

The correct answer is (b). Adie's syndrome occurs when the ciliary ganglion behind the eye is damaged from viral or bacterial infection. This may occur after an otherwise harmless URI. Without parasympathetic input to the eye, the pupil doesn't want to constrict at distance or near. With time (years, usually) the parasympathetic nerves grow back in. These nerves often grow "aberrantly," connecting too "strongly" to the iris constrictor muscles. This causes the iris to overconstrict and the pupil to stay small. This is called a "little old Adie's pupil."

14. When performing the swinging light test, which is the most important pupil response?
A. consensual response
B. indirect response
C. coerced response
D. slurred response

The correct answer is (a). The swinging light test is used to check the eye's overall ability to detect light by comparing the pupil size when shining a light in either eye. It works because the pupil will constrict in both the illuminated eye (a direct response) and also in the other eye (the consensual response). The other "responses" were made up.

15. Myasthenia gravis patients may have all of the following, except:
A. ptosis
B. thyroid dysfunction
C. chest tumor
D. dilated pupil

The correct answer is (d). Myasthenia gravis is a neuromuscular disorder that is characterized by easy fatigability. It often manifests with ocular findings, including drooping eyelid (ptosis) and double vision from extraocular muscle involvement. This condition does not involve smooth muscle so the iris is unaffected. Myasthenia gravis is also associated with thyroid dysfunction and 15% of patients with MG have a tumor of the thymus within the chest cavity.

16. What cranial nerve do the pupil constrictor fibers run through on their way to innervating the iris?
A. CN2
B. CN3
C. CN4
D. CN5

The correct answer is (b). The parasympathetic pupil constrictor nerves leave the Edinger-Westphal nucleus and travel with the third nerve as it exits the brainstem. In fact, many people with a third-nerve palsy will have a dilated or blown pupil. These pupil fibers run along the outside of the third nerve and are especially susceptible to damage from compressing lesions like tumor or aneurysm. An oculomotor nerve palsy with pupillary involvement is never a good sign.

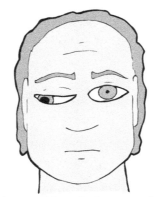

Third-nerve palsies make the eye turn "down and out" and give a blown pupil.

17. A patient complains of decreased temporal "side vision" in both eyes. They may have a lesion at the:
A. optic nerve
B. chiasm
C. optic tract
D. occipital lobe

CHAPTER 8: NEURO

The best answer (b). The fibers from the optic nerve cross at the chiasm, and lesions here knock out the side vision, causing a kind of "tunnel vision." Lesions further back cause congruent visual field defects that look the same in both eyes, especially moving back toward the occipital cortex. In other words, the further back in the brain you go, the more similar a visual field problem will look between the eyes.

18. Causes of diplopia include all, <u>except</u>:
A. stroke
B. decompensation
C. thyroid
D. thymus dysfunction

The best answer is (d). There are many causes for double vision such as stroke. Sometimes double vision is simply a decompensation of a pre-existing phoria (tendency for the eyes to wander) that happens with age. Thyroid dysfunction is a common cause of diplopia as well. Myasthenia gravis is another cause. Thymoma is associated with myasthenia gravis, but thymus dysfunction does not cause double vision by itself.

19. Sixth nerve palsy is most associated with:
A. aneurysm
B. pupil dilation
C. trauma
D. cranial pressure

The best answer is (d). Most nerve palsies are caused by vasculopathic problems such as diabetes and hypertension. Sixth nerve palsies are also associated with high intracranial pressure from pseudotumor cerebri. Third nerve palsies are associated with aneurysm and pupil dilation while fourth nerve palsy has many causes including trauma (the fourth nerve is long and skinny and easy to damage).

20. Sudden and complete vision loss may be caused by:
A. temporal arteritis
B. wet macular degeneration
C. cavernous sinus thrombosis
D. complete third nerve palsy

The best answer is (a). Temporal arteritis is an inflammatory condition involving the arteries of the head and neck. Arterial inflammation can lead to sudden blockage of the arteries around the eye and cause a central retinal artery occlusion or blockage of the arteries supplying the choroid. This may cause a sudden and drastic loss of vision. In contrast, wet macular degeneration may cause sudden distortion of central vision, but most of the peripheral vision would remain untouched. Cavernous sinus thrombosis may cause proptosis of the eye and affect most of the cranial nerves to the eye (CN3, CN4, CN6), but the optic nerve doesn't run through the cavernous sinus. As a result, this condition wouldn't cause sudden blindness. Finally, a third nerve palsy would cause major diplopia and pupil dilation but not vision loss.

21. New optic nerve swelling in a 55-year-old man is most likely caused by:
A. multiple sclerosis
B. ischemic optic neuropathy
C. giant cell arteritis
D. Cialis

The best answer is (b). There is a massive list of things that could cause monocular optic nerve swelling in our patients, but at this level of training you should be aware of three. In younger patients, the most common cause is optic neuritis. Optic neuritis is inflammation of the nerve, and while associated with multiple sclerosis, is not necessarily the same thing. In middle age, ION (ischemic optic neuropathy) is most common. This is an ischemic event that occurs at the optic disc that causes nerve swelling and an altitudinal visual defect (loss of the upper or lower vision). This

CHAPTER 8: NEURO

entity is associated with tight optic nerves, the so-called "disc at risk." The final entity you should keep on your radar is giant cell arteritis, which is also called temporal arteritis. This is an inflammatory condition of the blood vessels that occurs in elderly (typically 65+) that can cause many ischemic events around the eye. Erectile dysfunction medications like Cialis "may" be associated with optic nerve problems, but the causal relationship is not obvious. Most IONs occur in patients with vascular damage from age/hypertension, and these are the same people who might also need medications for ED.

22. Increased intracranial pressure can be caused by:
A. antibiotics
B. migraines
C. cycloplegia
D. diuretics

The best answer is (a). Pseudotumor cerebri occurs when the intracranial pressure (ICP) increases. This condition is often idiopathic in young women though several things may exacerbate it, including recent antibiotic use (especially tetracyclines), vitamin-A related acne medicines, and weight gain. Migraines or headache may be exacerbated by high intracranial pressure, but isn't the "cause" of pseudotumor. Cycloplegia is when we intentionally dilate eyes. Treatment for pseudotumor is often weight loss and oral diuretics such as Diamox.

23. A cavernous sinus tumor may affect all the cranial nerves, except:
A. CN 2
B. CN 3
C. CN 4
D. CN 5

The correct answer is (a). A lot of cranial nerves run through the cavernous sinus, including the nerves involved with eye movement

(3,4,6). Also, the first two divisions of CN 5 travel through the cavernous sinus, which means a lesion in the sinus can affect sensation of the upper half of the face. The optic nerve (CN2) doesn't run through the cavernous sinus at all, passing instead through the bony optic canal.

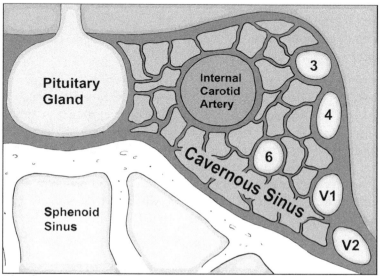

A lot of nerves run through the cavernous sinus. If your patient presents with multiple cranial nerve palsies, this is a likely place for their problem.

24. The pupil constricts with all, <u>except</u>:
A. light
B. accommodation
C. pilocarpine
D. atropine

The best answer is (d). The pupil constricts with light and accommodation (focusing on near objects). Pilocarpine is a topical drop that we use to constrict the pupils, often prior to laser procedures on the iris. Atropine is a long-acting dilating drop. It was discovered hundreds of years ago and derived from the belladona night shade plant. It was used by Victorian women to dilate their eyes as this was felt to make them look more seductive. The dilating effect of atropine is pretty long (a week), and so these women must have had a hell of a time seeing.

25. Risk factors for ischemic optic neuropathy include all of the following, except:
A. age
B. nocturnal hypotension
C. crowded optic nerve
D. glaucoma

The correct answer is (d). An ION causes severe nerve damage, often with an altitudinal (upper or lower) visual deficit. It tends to occur in middle-age people with vasculopathic risk factors like hypertension and diabetes. A common risk factor is the so-called "disc at risk." This is a tight optic nerve insertion, which can be seen as a small cup-to-disc ratio of 0.1. Also, low blood pressure at night seems to be a risk factor. Glaucoma, which usually causes a large cup-to-disc ratio, is not associated with ION.

26. Appropriate lab work for GCA (giant cell arteritis) includes all, except:
A. ESR
B. CRP
C. WBC
D. platelet count

The correct answer is (c). Giant cell arteritis (temporal arteritis) is an inflammation of the arteries around the head and eyes. It is related to polymyalgia rheumatica and can be potentially blinding if the ocular vessels are affected. Diagnosis is challenging, but the first step is bloodwork. ESR and CRP are the main inflammatory markers, but we also check platelet counts as they can elevate with the condition. WBC isn't typically affected by temporal arteritis.

27. When the optic nerve reaches the chiasm:
A. temporal fibers cross
B. nasal fibers cross
C. superior fibers cross
D. inferior fibers cross

The best answer is (b). At the optic chiasm, nasal nerve fibers cross. These fibers arise from the nasal retina. A lesion at the chiasm typically affects these crossing nasal fibers, causing the lateral side vision to knock out. If you find this hard to comprehend, just remember that a chiasm lesion, like an enlarging pituitary tumor, affects the side vision and gives you a kind of "tunnel vision."

28. Macular sparing of the vision occur when lesions in the:
A. chiasm
B. optic tract
C. occipital lobe
D. optic radiations

The best answer is (c). The occipital lobe is the final destination for the visual pathway. It is located at the back of the brain. The area is large, and most of it is dedicated to processing central vision. It is rare to have an occipital lesion large enough to knock out the entire central vision. Usually, the central "macular" vision remains intact.

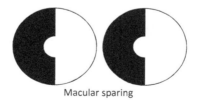
Macular sparing

29. If a person has lost vision in the right upper portion of their vision in both eyes, they may have a brain lesion in the:
A. right parietal lobe
B. right temporal lobe
C. left parietal lobe
D. left temporal lobe

The correct answer is (d). When trying to localize the location of a brain lesion, it is useful to think of the head as a giant eyeball and the back of the brain like the retina. Visual defects in the upper right vision correlate with brain lesions in the lower left brain (temporal lobe). These "pie-in-the-sky" field defects often map to the lower temporal lobe while "pie-on-the-floor" defects map to the upper parietal lobe.

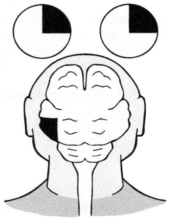

A right-upper vision defect maps out to a left-lower brain defect.

30. The more congruous (the same) a visual field deficit is, the more likely a lesion is located near the:
A. optic nerve
B. chiasm
C. lateral geniculate nucleus
D. occipital lobe

The correct answer is (d). In general, the more similar a visual field defect looks between the eyes, the closer the lesion is located to the occipital lobe. That's because the signals from each eye mix at the chiasm and become more intertwined as they travel to the occipital lobe at the back of the brain. An occipital lesion causes extremely similar deficits between the eyes, often with sparing of the macula.

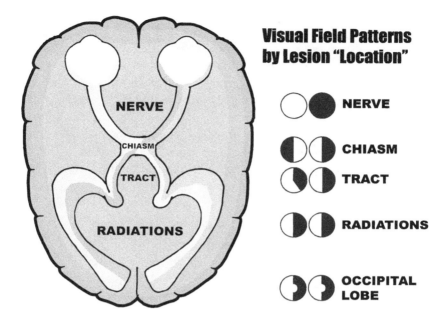

31. What double vision is most deadly?
A. binocular
B. monocular
C. trinocular
D. monocyclic

The correct answer is (a). Binocular diplopia implies a misalignment problem between the eyes. It can be caused by a number of scary things, including tumor. Monocular diplopia is double-images that occur only in a single eye and is often caused by astigmatism or cataract. Trinocular diplopia doesn't exist unless you have three eyes (or have been hit with a tricycle). Monocylic diplopia doesn't exist.

32. An advantage to stick-on prisms is that they:
A. are inexpensive
B. improve visual clarity
C. improve cosmesis
D. are easy to apply

CHAPTER 8: NEURO

The best answer is (a). Stick-on prisms are adhesive fresnel prisms that can be cut out and adhered to the surface of a patient's glasses. They are often used as a temporary cure for diplopia, as they are cheaper then getting prism ground into spectacles. They may also be used to help titrate prism correction or to insure the patient will tolerate the correction before making expensive prism spectacles. The downside is that stick-on prisms are unsightly and have ridges built into them that also decrease visual acuity. They can be difficult to apply, as the prism sticker must be cut out to fit the glasses and oriented correctly.

33. Pupil involvement with a third nerve palsy implies:
A. internal nerve ischemia
B. nerve compression
C. midbrain stroke
D. increased intracranial pressure

The best answer is (b). The parasympathetic pupil constricting fibers run along the outside of the third cranial nerve. Compressing lesions from the outside (such as a tumor or berry aneurysm) push on the nerve and can make the pupil dilate. A pupil-involving third nerve palsy is an ominous finding and always prompts a brain scan. Increased cranial pressure is associated more with sixth nerve palsy.

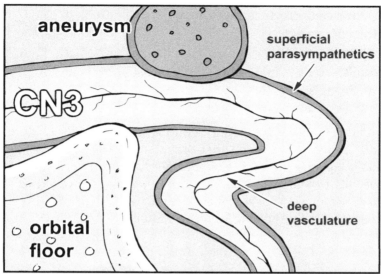

The parasympathetic "constrictor" fibers run along the surface of the third nerve. They are thus more susceptable to damage when compressing lesions from the outside impinge on the nerve.

34. What is <u>false</u> about optic neuritis?
A. patients often have decreased contrast sensitivity
B. patients often have problems with color vision
C. it is synonymous with multiple sclerosis
D. eye pain may get worse in hot tubs.

The correct answer is (c). Optic neuritis is an inflammation of the optic nerve, most common in young people. These patients often have problems with their color vision and decreased contrast sensitivity (though few eye doctors bother to check contrast). They may also have central or centrocecal visual field deficits. Many of these patients have eye pain with movement, as the irritated optic nerve is shifted when the eyes move. One uncommon finding is the Uhthoff's phenomenon. This is eye pain exacerbated by heat, such as bathing or exercise. While optic neuritis is a common prequel to multiple sclerosis, its presence doesn't guarantee the disease. Not all cases of optic neuritis develop MS, and not all patients with MS ever have an episode of optic neuritis. A more predictable indicator of future MS is the presence of demyelinating lesions on MRI.

CHAPTER 8: NEURO

35. Optic neuritis is treated with:
A. topical steroids
B. injected steroids
C. oral steroids
D. IV steroids

The correct answer is (d). Optic neuritis is treated with IV steroids. Oddly, studies have found that oral steroids like prednisone may actually <u>increase</u> the chance of optic neuritis recurrence. We usually leave this treatment in the hands of neurology, however, as they usually want an MRI and may want to use interferon (Avonex) medicines if demyelinating lesions are found.

CHAPTER 9
OPTICS

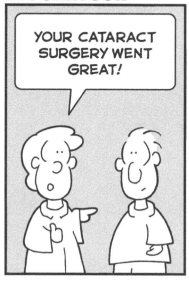
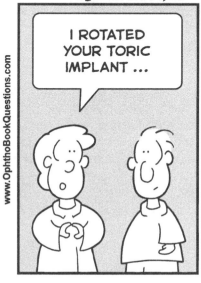
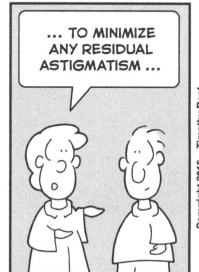
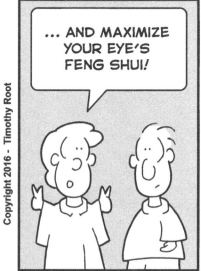

OPTICS

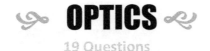

19 Questions

1. Measures of visual acuity include all, <u>except</u>:
A. Snellen
B. logMAR
C. Jaeger
D. Humphrey

The correct answer is (d). The Humphrey visual field machine is used to check peripheral vision - it does not measure visual acuity. The Snellen chart, however, is the eye chart that is most commonly used in the office. This is the chart with the large E at the top with 20/20 Snellen acuity considered normal. The logMAR chart is a more accurate logarithmic chart that uses numbers. It is primarily used in research studies requiring a more accurate vision measurement. The Jaeger scale is used for measuring near vision and is recorded as J1, J2, etc.

2. If a patient reads the eye chart better when looking through a pinhole occluder, then this implies they have a problem with their:
A. accommodation
B. refraction
C. contrast
D. convergence

The correct answer is (b). The pinhole occluder is used during an eye exam to see if a patient has a problem with refraction - i.e., does a patient need to get glasses or need their current spectacles updated. The pinhole works by converting the eye from a "lens focusing camera" to a "pinhole camera." Pinhole cameras are always in perfect focus because light coming off an object can only enter the camera through a single entry point before striking the film/retina. If a patient sees better through the pinhole, this implies their "lens system" needs tweaking to bring it up to speed.

Accommodation is the process by which the eye focuses at near objects. Contrast is the ability to differentiate between subtle shades of color, while convergence is the ability for the eyes to cross.

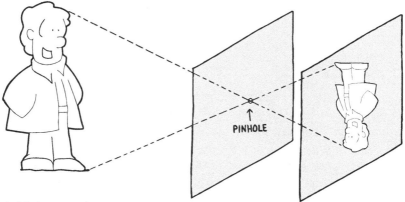

A pinhole camera does not need to be focused. Light bouncing off a subject can only enter the camera through the small hole and strike a single spot on the film behind.

3. What must an emmetropic eye do to read a book?
A. accommodate
B. diverge
C. myope
D. conjugate

The answer is (a). An "emmetropic" eye is merely an eye that is in perfect focus for distance vision. This is in contrast to a myopic (nearsighted) eye that is focused for near and a hyperopic (farsighted) eye that isn't focused for <u>any</u> distance. For an emmetropic eye to read, the eye must accommodate. This is when the lens inside the eye becomes rounder and increases the refractive power of the eye to view near objects clearly. Children have flexible lenses inside their eye and can accommodate easily. When we age, however, the lens stiffens and accommodation becomes difficult, necessitating the need for reading glasses. Divergence is when the eyes turn outward. "Myope" is just a noun to describe a nearsighted person, and isn't a verb at all (in other words, you can't myope something). Finally, *conjugate* is a good descriptor for *the other eye* as in "the other eye had normal conjugate movements."

4. Nearsighted eyes tend to be:
A. larger
B. shorter
C. thicker
D. attractive

The best answer is (a). Nearsighted eyes tend to be large and longer than normal. This causes images to focus, not on the retina, but in the vitreous gel in front of the retina. The other answers are incorrect. Myopia doesn't make the eye "thicker," though there are conditions such as nanophthalmos that show thickening of the scleral wall. Large eyes are, at least in Western culture, a sign of beauty, but apparent eye size is more a result of the size of the palpebral fissure between the eyelids.

5. With accommodation:
A. zonules relax and the lens rounds
B. zonules tighten and the lens rounds
C. zonules relax and the lens flattens
D. zonules tighten and the lens flattens

The best answer is (a). Accommodation is the act of focusing on near objects. The eye accomplishes this by contracting the round ciliary body/muscle, located behind the iris. When this muscle contracts, it squeezes inwards like a sphincter. This action relaxes the zonules that suspend the lens, allowing the lens to become rounder. A round lens is a more powerful lens, which is needed to focus on near objects.

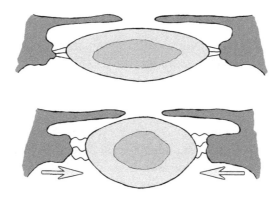

With accommodation, the ciliary body contracts, zonules relax, and the lens becomes rounder (more powerful).

6. Astigmatism can be all, <u>except</u>:
A. corneal
B. lenticular
C. vitreal
D. irregular

The best answer is (c). Astigmatism is usually described as curvature to the eye such that the horizontal and vertical curvatures are different. In other words, instead of the eye being round like a basketball, the eye is shaped more like a football. This astigmatism is often in the cornea, but can also be in the lens. This is called lenticular astigmatism. Irregular astigmatism is when the eye curvature is even more irregular, such as from scarring or ectatic disorders such as keratoconus.

7. Convert +1.00 +2.00 x 180 into minus cylinder.
A. -1.00 -2.00 x 090
B. -1.00 -2.00 x 180
C. +3.00 -2.00 x 090
D. +3.00 -2.00 x 180

The correct answer is (c). A prescription can be measured and documented in either "plus" or "minus" format. To convert from plus cylinder into minus (and vice versa), you must do three things:

CHAPTER 9: OPTICS

1. Add the cylinder power to the spherical power (you remember how to add negative numbers, right?)
2. Change the sign (positive or negative) of the cylinder power
3. Change the axis by 90 degrees.

Optometrists love working in minus cylinder, because that's how glasses are made. Ophthalmologists love working in plus cylinder, because it is easier to conceptualize (and helpful when making astigmatic incisions in the cornea). Neither method is better: they are mathematically the same. Watch my optics lecture at www.OphthoBook.com if you are confused.

8. Hyperopic eyes are in focus for:
A. distance
B. near
C. both
D. neither

The best answer is (d). Farsighted, hyperopic eyes aren't really in focus for near OR distance. These patients complain of more near problems, however.

9. What is the spherical equivalent of: +1.50 +3.00 x 180
A. +1.50
B. +3.00
C. +3.75
D.+ 4.50

The correct answer is (b). Spherical equivalent is calculated by taking half of the cylinder power and adding this to the spherical power. This might be useful in a patient with astigmatism who you want to fit with a regular (non-toric) contact. Alternatively, a farsighted patient might be able to drive with cheap, over-the-counter reading glasses if they are the correct spherical equivalent.

10. Your patient wears a +5.00 glasses prescription. The patient is interested in contacts, as the thick glasses are hurting the bridge of his nose. His final contact lens prescription will likely be:
A. +4.50
B. +4.75
C. +5.00
D. +5.25

The best answer is (d). A contact lens requires more "plus" power than glasses, because they sit on the eyeball itself. This is a hard concept to grasp, but let me explain. Imagine you were examining Pinocchio. Pinocchio has a very long nose and his glasses sit on the end of this honker. He is farsighted, and wears +4.00 glasses that allow images to focus on the surface of his retina. Now imagine, the "blue fairy" shows up and shrinks his nose, bringing his spectacles closer to the eye. The "focal point" of his glasses moves in synchrony with his glasses, so images now focus behind his eye! That's no good! In order to pull the focal point "forward," Pinocchio needs a stronger glasses prescription with a shorter focal point. Now, if he gets a nose job and brings his glasses even closer to his eyes (shoving them onto his eyes like contacts), the same problem will occur. He now requires a stronger lens to focus on the nearby retina. Therefore, contacts must have more (+) power to be equivalent to glasses.

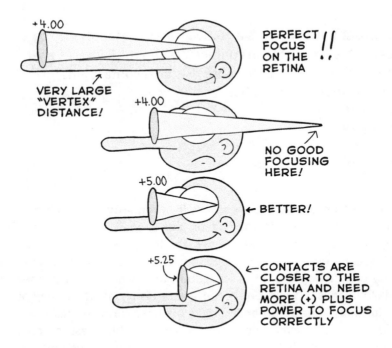

11. Where does the majority of light refraction <u>actually</u> occur?
A. tears
B. cornea
C. aqueous
D. lens

The correct answer is (a). Light bends when passing through an interface of variable density. In the eye, the density gradient between air and the tear film is highest so the tear-air interface is where the majority of light refraction occurs.

12. Diopter is a measurement of:
A. refractive power
B. prism power
C. both
D. neither

The best answer is (c). A diopter is a measurement of both refraction <u>and</u> prism power. With refraction, a diopter is used to describe the focal point of a lens. A 1 diopter lens focuses light at one meter while a 3 diopter lens has a focal point of one-third meter. This explains why many reading glasses have a power of +3.00 - many people prefer to hold books 33 cm away from their eyes. Prism diopters are used to describe the bending of light. This measurement is referenced at one meter. If you shoot a laser beam through a prism so that it strikes a wall one meter away, the light will be deviated 1 cm for every prism diopter in the lens.

13. An <u>inappropriate</u> prism diopter adjustment to fix double vision would be:
A. 2 BO, 2 BO
B. 3 BI, 1 BI
C. 4 BU, 1 BD
D. 2 BI, 2 BO

The best answer is (d). Prism is documented in regards to the "base," which refers to the thick part of the prism glass. This base can be pointed inward, outward, up, or down. If someone was cross-eyed, for instance, you might use bilateral "base-out" prisms to "pull" the eyes outwards. If your patient had a vertical deviation, you might use a base-up prism to correct this. Alternatively, you might split the prism into a base-up in one eye, and a base-down in the other eye to keep the glasses from being too heavy or lopsided. The last answer doesn't make sense: a base-out prism on the right eye would "pull" the right eye to the right, while a base-in prism on the left eye would <u>also</u> pull to the right. This wouldn't fix any eye alignment issues, but would instead force the patient to turn his or her head to see straight.

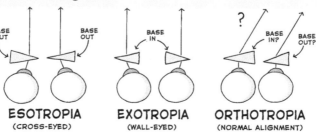

CHAPTER 9: OPTICS

14. "No line" bifocal glasses are also known as:
A. transitional
B. progressive
C. gradual
D. executive

The best answer is (b). Progressive bifocals have no visible line on them, but get stronger the further down you look. Transitional glasses darken when exposed to UV light. There is no such thing as "gradual" glasses. Executive top is a type bifocal with a straight-top edge.

15. A +4 diopter lens focuses light at:
A. 100 cm
B. 80 cm
C. 25 cm
D. 20 cm

The best answer here is (c). The dioptric power of a lens tells us where that lenses focal point is. This focal point is the reciprocal of the diopter power. For example, a 1 diopter lens focuses at one meter, while a 2 diopter lens focuses at one-half meter (50 cm). A 4 diopter lens focuses at one-fourth of a meter, or 25 cm.

16. The cornea is responsible for what percentage of overall refraction in the eye:
A. 1/3
B. 1/4
C. 1/2
D. 2/3

The best answer is (d). The cornea is a fixed lens and does the majority of refraction (light-bending) in the eye. Overall, the eye has about 60 diopters of power, with the cornea responsible for about 40 diopters of this total.

17. If stranded on a deserted island, who would have the easiest time starting a fire with their glasses?
A. myope
B. hyperope
C. emmetrope
D. triope

The best answer here is (b). Hyperopic (farsighted) eyes are weak and short. They require "plus" power lenses in their glasses to see. These plus convex lenses work just like a magnifying glass, and can be used to focus light from the sun to start small fires. Nearsighted people wear minus, concave lenses that can't be used to focus the sun. Emmetropes have no refractive error and therefore do not typically wear glasses. Triopes are small shrimp-like organisms that propagate in mud puddles after a desert rainfall. You can grow them at home, just like sea monkeys.

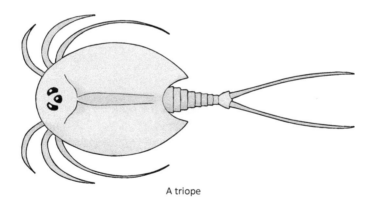

A triope

18. When fitting someone for contacts, important measurements might include all, except:
A. vertex distance
B. axial length
C. corneal curvature
D. corneal diameter

CHAPTER 9: OPTICS

The best answer is (b). Contacts are a bit more complicated than glasses, as a contact must fit properly or risk discomfort and corneal irritation. Contact prescriptions contain more measurements than glasses. One of these measurements is the "base curve" that describes the steepness of the contact. They also contain a diameter measurement as well. While we don't typically need to measure the patient's corneal diameter (it's usually around 11-12 mm for everyone) we DEFINITELY don't measure the patient's axial length. This measurement, the distance from the cornea to the retina, is really only needed when calculating cataract implants (and the occasional oddball optics question). The vertex distance is the distance from the eye to the back of a person's glasses. People with large noses have a larger vertex distance and therefore may require a larger difference in contact lens power. This is a really hard question, so don't worry if you missed it!

19. RGP contacts are
A. hard
B. soft
C. extended wear
D. colored

The correct answer is (a). RGP stands for rigid gas permeable and is what we commonly call "hard contacts." This type of contact is rigid, but still permeable to oxygen, unlike the old PMMA (Plexiglas) contacts of the '70s.

CHAPTER 10
PEDIATRICS

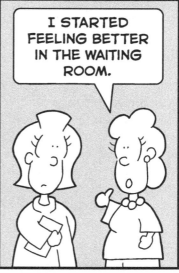
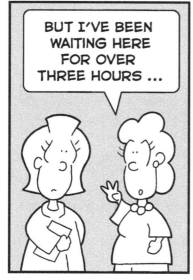
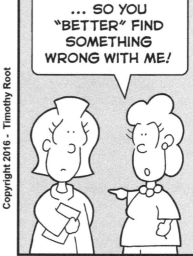

PEDIATRICS

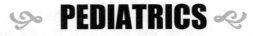
23 Questions

1. A white pupil can be caused by all, <u>except</u>:
A. retinal detachment
B. ROP
C. tumor
D. ARDS

The best answer is (d). Pupil examination is part of every well-baby exam. The causes for a white pupil are all quite serious. The classic one we fear is retinoblastoma, a tumor of the photoreceptors inside the eye. This tumor can spread and kill the child if unrecognized. Retinopathy of prematurity (ROP) can cause retinal detachments and give a white pupil, as can a congenital cataract. ARDS (acute respiratory distress syndrome) is unrelated to the eye, though it does increase the risk of ROP in the premature neonate.

2. A large angle esotropia might be corrected with any of the following surgery techniques, <u>except</u>?
A. medial rectus recession
B. lateral rectus resection
C. medial rectus detachment
D. adjustable sutures

The best answer here is (c). When the eyes are crossed (esotropia) surgical manipulation of the medial and lateral rectus muscles can help straighten them. Either the lateral rectus muscles can be tightened (resection) or the inner medial muscles can be loosened (recession). Some strabismus doctors use adjustable sutures to help titrate the correction after surgery, though this is best done on adults who can cooperate during their post-operative exams. One complication of muscle surgery is to "drop" or lose the muscle during surgery. Safety stitches are tied to the muscle prior to cutting it so that this doesn't happen. If the muscle is lost behind the eye, this "detachment" will result in even more eye movement problems.

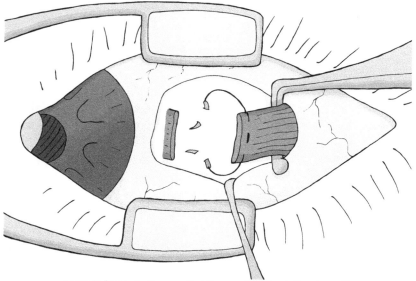

A muscle "recession" means that the muscle action is "weakened" by sewing it behind its original insertion point.

3. Tearing in an infant can be caused by all, <u>except</u>:
A. nasolacrimal duct obstruction
B. enlarged lacrimal glands
C. glaucoma
D. Hasner valve obstruction

The best answer here is (b). The most common cause of excess tearing in a child is nasolacrimal duct obstruction. This is when the pathway of tear drainage into the nose is blocked. This occurs because of an incomplete opening of the valve of Hasner inside the nose and is often treated with massage, probing, and temporary stent placement. Congenital glaucoma causes eyeball enlargement and excess tearing. Enlargement of the lacrimal gland, from inflammation (dacryoadenitis) or tumor, is very rare and causes swelling of the upper eyelid or eyeball displacement.

CHAPTER 10: PEDIATRICS

4. If probing the nasolacrimal system fails to keep the duct flowing, the next step may be:
A. Crawford tube
B. Jones tube
C. Foley tube
D. VP shunt

The best answer here is (a). To keep the nasolacrimal duct open, a thin stent called a Crawford tube is threaded through this drainage pathway and tied off inside the nose. This tube is left for several months before being removed. Hopefully the tear pathway will remain open after this. If not, a DCR surgery may be attempted. With permanent blockage of the nasolacrimal duct system, a Jones Tube may have to be placed. This is a glass tube placed in the corner of the eyelid that drains tears directly through nasal bones into the nose. A Foley catheter is used for urinary drainage and a ventriculoperitoneal shunt drains fluid from the brain into the abdominal cavity.

5. Indicators for potential retinopathy in a newborn include:
A. low birth weight
B. hypoxia issues
C. prematurity
D. all of the above

The best answer here is (d). Retinopathy of prematurity occurs when a child is born before their retinal vasculature has fully formed. Forced to "work" before it is ready, the retinal cells become hungry for oxygen and began to grow abnormal "neovascular" blood vessels. These abnormal vessels create scarring, bleeding, traction, and can even cause a retinal detachment. Risk factors for ROP include prematurity (less than 32 weeks gestation), hypoxia problems (including exposure to high levels of oxygen), low birth weight (less than 1250 grams), and any severe illness. The treatment is similar to the treatment for neovascular diabetic retinopathy - PRP laser (to decrease "hungry" retinal tissue production of VEGF) and treating any retinal detachments with laser or surgery.

6. With conjunctivitis, what group is most likely to have a bacterial infection?
A. adults
B. elderly
C. children
D. dog owners

The best answer is (c). With adults, the most likely cause of conjunctivitis is viral infection. This is not true with children, who are more likely to have a bacterial eye infection. I am not aware of any differences with elderly or dog owners, though the latter tend to be nice people.

7. The <u>worst</u> indicator of an infant's actual ability to "see" is:
A. pupil constriction
B. blinking to light
C. fixing and following objects
D. optokinetic response

The best answer here is (a). The pupil response only measures the ability for the eye to detect light (and the integrity of the pupillary pathway in the front part of the brain). Some unfortunate children are born with "cortical blindness" where the connections to the occipital cortex are not formed. Their pupils constrict but they cannot "see" anything. This can be tested using VEP (visual evoked potential) where electrodes are placed on the back of the head to measure the signal at the occipital lobe when lights are projected into the eyes. If a child can blink to light or follow objects, then you know that they can see, since this indicates that they are responding to their environment. The optokinetic drum can be useful as well. This is a small barrel with striped lines that you spin in front of the child. As their eyes track the barrel lines you'll see their eyes jerk rhythmically. A good OKN response usually indicates that vision is at least 20/200.

CHAPTER 10: PEDIATRICS

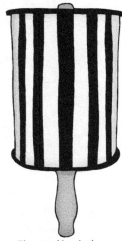

The optokinetic drum

8. Amblyopia can be caused from all these conditions, <u>except</u>:
A. low birth weight
B. astigmatism
C. ptosis
D. cataract

> The best answer is (a). Amblyopia is an extremely common cause of poor vision, and is secondary to incomplete formation of the visual nervous system at a young age. Anything that decreases the vision in one eye will cause the "wiring" in the good eye to predominate, turning the poorer eye into a "lazy" eye that never sees as well. Common causes for amblyopia are strabismus (eyes out of alignment), refractive imbalance (including large amounts of monocular astigmatism), and blockages of the visual pathway (cataract, drooping eyelid). Low birth weight increases the risk of ROP, not amblyopia.

9. Amblyopia can be treated with all, <u>except</u>:
A. drops
B. patching
C. glasses
D. pills

The correct answer is (d). Amblyopia, also called "lazy eye," occurs from incomplete "wiring" of the visual pathway from the eyeball to the occipital lobe. The main treatment for this condition is to patch the good eye to allow the weaker eye a chance to form properly. Patching is challenging in this age group. Occasionally, chemical patching of the strong eye with a strong dilating drop like atropine can be used. Correction of any existing refractive error (like hyperopia) is also extremely important. There aren't any pills that will help with this condition (other than Xanax, for the flustered parents who have been battling their child to wear the patch).

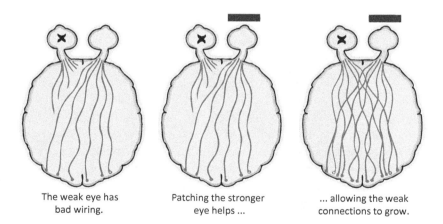

The weak eye has bad wiring.

Patching the stronger eye helps ...

... allowing the weak connections to grow.

10. The number one cause of leukocoria in an infant is:
A. retinoblastoma
B. congenital cataract
C. retinopathy of prematurity
D. asteroid hyalosis

CHAPTER 10: PEDIATRICS

The best answer here is (b). Leukocoria, a white pupil, is an ominous sign in a child, as there are many bad things that can cause this. The most common is likely congenital cataract. If born with a cataract, this needs to be treated within the first few months of life as it will cause a dense sensory amblyopia (lazy eye). Retinoblastoma is a very dangerous tumor of the photoreceptors inside the eye that causes a large white mass. This is rare, with only 400 cases a year in the US, but may potentially become life-threatening. ROP can lead to a white pupil if it causes a retinal detachment. There are other causes of leukocoria such as infection, PHPV, and Coat's disease of the retina. Asteroid hyalosis isn't one of them, however, as this is a finding we see in older patients where they form harmless white calcium soap deposits in their eye that look like little asteroids floating in space.

11. Rhythmic movements of the eyes are known as:
A. saccades
B. nystagmus
C. vestibular jerks
D. ocular bobbing

The correct answer is (b). Nystagmus is a rhythmic, to-and-fro movement of the eyes. This movement usually consists of a fast eye movement in one direction, followed by a slower movement in the other. The nystagmus is named after the fast phase, such that an up-beating nystagmus would have the fast phase going upwards. There are several causes for nystagmus. Some are congenital, such as *congenital motor nystagmus*. Sensory nystagmus is an acquired problem in children who have very poor vision at a young age, when the visual system is still forming. The other answers are incorrect. A saccade is the large, ballistic movement of the eye when you look back and forth at different objects. Ocular bobbing is an extremely rare, downward nystagmus that is associated with ocular paralysis and is found with major brain damage. "Vestibular jerks" is a made up term that could be used to describe arrogant ENT doctors.

12. Latent nystagmus get worse when:
A. covering one eye
B. looking in a certain direction
C. fogging the vision
D. you're intoxicated

The correct answer is (a). Latent nystagmus are quick movements (nystagmus) of the eyes that only occur when you cover one eye. These nystagmus are sometimes hard to pick up until you start checking vision: as soon as you occlude one eye in the phoropter, your patient's vision goes to pot. To offset this, we typically "fog" the patient by placing the wrong prescription in front of the occluded eye to blur it without completely blocking the vision. Nystagmus that become worse when looking to the side is usually called "end-point nystagmus." This is a normal finding, but may be more pronounced when tired, medicated, or intoxicated.

13. The null point is:
A. direction of minimal nystagmus
B. prime tenant of the scientific method
C. focal point of a lens system
D. spot of minimal chromatic aberration

The correct answer is (a). Many children with nystagmus (jerking movement of the eyes) have a direction of gaze where the eye jerking is minimal, giving them the best uninterrupted vision. This point is called the "null point." If straight ahead, great - but often, this direction occurs when looking off to the side. The child may adopt an unatural head turn to keep them in the null point. Occasionally we'll put prisms in glasses (or perform surgery) to deviate the eyes so they are more often in the null point, thereby fixing the head turn. As for the other answers: the null hypothesis is the key tenant of the scientific method. The nodal point is a theoretical central point of the eyes lens system and is located at the back of the lens. Cataract opacities closer to this nodal point (such as PSC cataracts) seem to cause more visual complaints than ones further anterior.

CHAPTER 10: PEDIATRICS

14. Children with new nystagmus get an MRI because of potential:
A. optic nerve glioma
B. agenesis of the corpus callosum
C. brainstem lesions
D. arnold chiari malformation

While all these conditions <u>could</u> cause eye problems, the best answer is (a). An optic nerve glioma is a tumor that forms in the optic nerve or chiasm behind the eye. It usually presents in childhood and is associated with neurofibromatosis 1. It may have no presenting symptoms other than decreased vision, though later stages show proptosis and optic nerve edema. Unfortunately, children can't always tell us they are having visual difficulties, and the only presenting symptom may be sensory nystagmus. Most cases of acquired nystagmus warrant imaging, though there are some types of nystagmus syndromes (like spasmus nutans) that are self-limited. The other conditions will also be detected with an MRI, but are often associated with other problems besides nystagmus. For example, brainstem lesions may cause alignment problems because of involvement of the cranial nerve nuclei. This was a hard question.

15. Young children are often dilated with cyclopentolate because:
A. they have strong accommodation
B. children dilate poorly
C. there are less systemic side effects
D. it stings less

The best answer is (a). Children have very strong ciliary muscles that allow them to accommodate strongly. In fact, they can accommodate so strongly that they can focus on letters only a few inches in front of their eyes. This makes it extremely difficult to check them for glasses as they accommodate and strain their way through the eye exam. We normally dilate our adult patients with tropicamide to paralyze the ciliary muscle, but kids often require a stronger cycloplegic agent like cyclopentolate. Most kids under 10 (or who have a confusing prescription) get a "cyclo refraction." Unfortunately, this lengthens the child's visit time as we have to refract them again after they are dilated.

16. All of the following may cause pseudoesotropia, <u>except</u>:
A. telecanthus
B. Asian race
C. epicanthal fold
D. small pupillary distance

The best answer is (a). Pseudoesotropia is the illusion of having crossed eyes, even though the eyes are in good alignment. Pseudoesotropia is common in young children and Asians, who have a medial epicanthal fold that covers much of the nasal sclera. Telecanthus is a cosmetic finding where the distance between the medial canthi (inner corners of the eyelid) is wider than average. This tends to make the eyes look wider apart and can give the illusion of <u>exo</u>tropia. A good example of telecanthus is Jackie Onassis (JFK's widow).

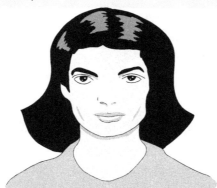

Telecanthus is wide-set eyes but normal bony anatomy on CT scan.

17. What does the Hirschberg test detect?
A. amblyopia
B. strabismus
C. hyperopia
D. pupil response

The correct answer is (b). The Hirschberg test, also known as the corneal light test, is a simple method to estimate ocular alignment problems in children (who might not cooperate with more traditional measurements like the cover-uncover test). It involves shooting a penlight at the child's eyes and examining the location of the corneal light reflection in relationship to the child's pupils. A normal corneal reflection should be directly over the pupils. For every millimeter that the reflection is deviated, this is said to correspond to 15 prism diopters of misalignment.

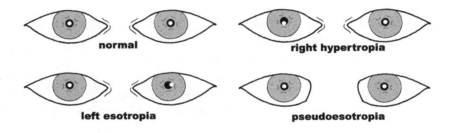

18. What is Crede prophylaxis?
A. neonatal antibiotics
B. amblyopia screening
C. panretinal photocoagulation
D. a rock band

The correct answer is (a). All newborns, at least in the US, receive antibiotic eye treatment after birth to decrease the chance of neonatal gonorrhea and chlamydia. This is called Crede prophylaxis. It is named after Dr. Carl Crede, who started this trend in 1881. Back then, however, he used silver nitrate, which is no longer available. In the US, we use erythromycin ointment. In some developing countries, povidone iodine is used instead to good effect, as it is effective and even cheaper.

19. A positive optokinetic response implies the child has vision that is at least:
A. 20/30
B. 20/50
C. 20/200
D. hand motion

The best answer is (c). The optokinetic drum is a handheld spinning barrel with white and black stripes painted on it. The barrel is held in front of the patient and slowly turned. Our eyes have a tendency to track objects and you will see the patient's eyes move and refixate on the lines as they go past. This response is useful in some children and for adults who cannot communicate (or for those who are malingering and say they are blind). If a patient has a normal optokinetic response to the drum, they are usually considered to have 20/200 vision or better.

20. The least appropriate way to check vision in children would be via:
A. Snellen chart
B. object tracking
C. tumbling E chart
D. picture optotypes

The best answer is (c). There are many ways to check and to document a child's vision. With newborns, we may only get a BTL (blink to light) response but soon we can document F&F (fixes and follows), as the child becomes interested in the surrounding world. The next progression is the ability to recognize picture optotypes. These are eye charts in which the letters have been replaced by pictures of flowers, horses, birthday cakes, etc. By the time kids reach kindergarten, they usually know their letters, and the Snellen chart can be attempted. The tumbling E chart is similar to the standard eye chart, except the letters have been replaced by the letter E oriented in different directions. This is helpful for illiterate or mute patients as they can orient their fingers in the same direction as the letter and show this to the examiner. This chart is also useful for foreign patients who don't use a western alphabet (Chinese). The tumbling E is hard to explain to a child. Any kid smart enough to respond correctly to this chart probably knows their alphabet already, and would do better with the Snellen or picture chart.

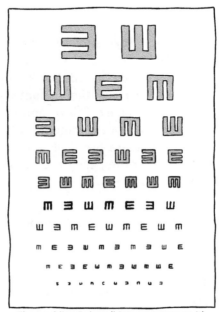

The tumbling E chart (hint: we never use it)

21. A child with accommodative esotropia might benefit from what type of glasses?
A. plus sphere
B. minus sphere
C. plus cylinder
D. minus cylinder

The best answer is (a). Accommodative esotropia occurs when a child's eyes cross when they accommodate. Let me explain. The eye muscles are yoked, so that when we focus on near objects, our ciliary body muscle accommodates (focuses the lens) and our rectus muscles turn the eyes inward toward the nose (crossed eyes). This is normal and is required for close-up vision. However, many children are born hyperopic (farsighted). Children have strong ciliary body muscles and are able to overcome farsightedness by accommodating strongly all the time. Unfortunately, this may also cause their eyes to cross all the time. We can give these children glasses to fix their hyperopia. This takes the strain off their ciliary muscle and allows their eyes to "relax." This may also decrease or eliminate their esotropia.

22. Retinoscopy is used to detect:
A. tropia
B. phoria
C. leukocoria
D. refraction

The best answer is (d). Retinoscopy is used to check refraction by examining how the red reflex looks when different lenses are held in front of the eye. This is helpful in preverbal children who can't be refracted at the phoropter. We also use it on adult patients who can't communicate well or who need to be examined while under anesthesia. It is also helpful for detecting astigmatism, and may be used concurrently with a normal refraction. Retinoscopy is one of the harder skills to learn as a young doctor/technician but it is an invaluable one if you work in the field. To learn the details, you may want to watch my retinoscopy lecture online, though this may be a little advanced for new students.

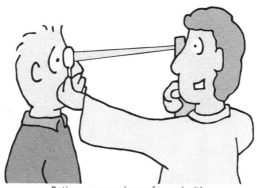

Retinoscopy can be performed with loose lenses, or at the phoropter.

CHAPTER 10: PEDIATRICS

23. When should congenital cataracts be operated on?
A. infancy
B. toddlerhood
C. early teenage years
D. late teenage years

The correct answer is (a). A congenital cataract is extremely amblyogenic for an infant, and they will quickly develop a "lazy eye." For this reason, congenital cataracts are removed early, usually within the first few months of life. Children's eyes are still growing at this age, however, and they tend to have extreme inflammatory responses. An implant is therefore not inserted until later. To improve vision, children wear aphakic glasses (if both eyes were operated on) or a contact lens (if one eye was operated on). As you can imagine, contacts are a major pain for parents.

CHAPTER 11
RETINA

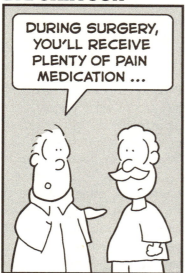
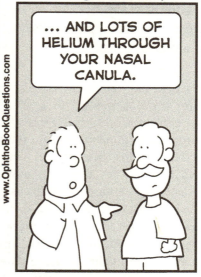
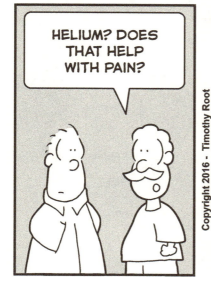
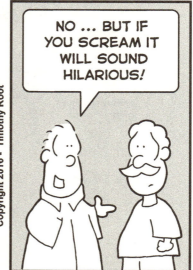

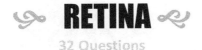

RETINA
32 Questions

1. Flashes and floaters are usually caused by:
A. vitreous detachment
B. endophthalmitis
C. ciliary body inflammation
D. aqueous cells

The best answer is (a). Flashes and floaters usually occur from a vitreous detachment. This is when the vitreous gel in the back of the eye contracts with age. As the vitreous peels off of the retina, it irritates the retina and causes flashing lights in the peripheral vision. Cellular debris at the gel interface causes floaters. Vitreous detachments are common and are the main cause of retinal detachment. Endophthalmitis is an infection inside the eye that causes floaters and rapidly decreasing vision. Endophthalmitis is rare, most often occuring after surgery or trauma. Ciliary body inflammation (uveitis) causes light sensitivity, as the ciliary muscle "spasms" with light exposure. The aqueous fluid is too far anterior in the visual pathway to produce discernible floaters.

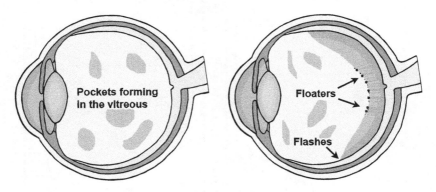

Vitreous liquification causes the jelly to contract, leading to floaters and flashing lights.

2. A Weiss ring is:
A. a ring of copper deposition
B. a ring of iron deposition
C. the edge of the retina
D. vitreous debris

The best answer is (d). A Weiss ring occurs after a vitreous detachment. When the vitreous gel contracts inside the eye, it peels off the surface of the retina. The vitreous is firmly adherent to the optic nerve. As the vitreous peels off the nerve, a circular ring of cellular debris will come off as well. This Weiss ring can be seen floating inside the eye at the vitreous interface. Patients sometimes describe seeing a large, oval floater in their vision. A Kayser-Fleischer ring occurs when the liver can't process copper; a green copper ring may form at the edge of the cornea. A Fleischer line is an iron line seen on the cornea that is usually a sign of dry eye or an incomplete blink. The edge of the retina is called the ora serrata.

3. A patient complains of losing vision in their left eye. The patient tells you that "everything below and to the right near my nose" looks blurry. You suspect a retinal detachment in what quadrant of the left eye?
A. superior-temporal
B. superior-nasal
C. inferior-temporal
D. inferior-nasal

The best answer is (a). The patient is describing vision problems in the inferior-nasal quadrant of their left eye. The retina is oriented inversely to what the patient sees. Therefore, the patient's retinal problem is in the superior-temporal quadrant, a common location for a retinal tear. If small, superior retinal breaks are more amenable to repair. Gas floats, so pneumatic retinopexy (injecting a bubble into the eye to tamponade the retina into position) only works on these superior breaks.

4. The most common retina test ordered is the:
A. FA
B. autofluorescence
C. ERG
D. OCT

The best answer is (d). OCT (optical coherence tomography) is the most common retina test we order. It works similar to ultrasound but uses light waves instead of sound waves to create a map of the retina surface. This is great for picking up wet macular degeneration, macular edema after surgery, and CSME (clinically significant macular edema) from diabetes. FA is the abbreviation for fluorescein angiogram. This involves injecting yellow fluorescein dye into the arm and taking serial photographs of the retina as this dye perfuses the retinal vasculature. ERG stands for electroretinogram. ERG measures the electric signal the retina generates when stimulated by light (like measuring an EKG of the heart), and is useful for diagnosing rod/cone dystrophies and retinitis pigmentosa. This is a rare test, usually performed at larger, teaching hospitals. Autofluorescence is an uncommon photographic technique that uses lens filters to look at structures in the retina. It can be useful for examining optic nerve head drusen and other structures in the eye that are naturally fluorescent.

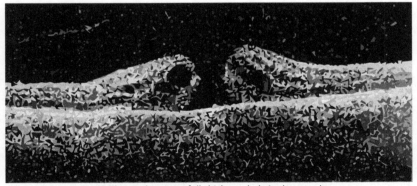

An OCT scan showing a full-thickness hole in the macula.

5. A positive Shafer sign suggests:
A. narrow angles
B. retinal detachment
C. esotropia
D. myasthenia gravis

The best answer here is (b). A positive Shafer sign is pigmented debris in the vitreous that occurs after a retinal break. It is seen as "tobacco dust" floating behind the lens during the slit-lamp exam. This pigment comes from the RPE (retinal pigmented epithelium) that lays under the retina. This pigment can travel through a retinal break to float in the vitreous. The other answers are incorrect, though answer (a) is close. We often use gonioscopy to examine patients with narrow angle glaucoma. We use a *Shaffer scale* to describe how tight this angle looks. A " Shaffer 4" means the angle is wide open, with "Shaffer 1" angles being at risk for having an acute glaucoma attack.

6. A sudden, complete loss of vision is most likely a:
A. retinal detachment
B. CRAO
C. wet macular degeneration
D. acute glaucoma

The best answer is (b). A CRAO (central retinal artery occlusion) occurs when the main artery that supplies the retina becomes blocked suddenly. This makes the vision blank out rapidly, and may lead to permanent retinal damage within hours if the blockage doesn't open up. The other answers are incorrect. Retinal detachments can proceed rapidly, but are usually preceded with vision loss in the peripheral vision first and have a flash/floater prodrome. Wet macular degeneration can cause a rapid decrease in central vision but doesn't affect the peripheral vision. Acute glaucoma can cause extreme eye pain and blurry vision, but not complete vision loss until significant nerve damage has occurred.

CHAPTER 11: RETINA

7. Widespread intraretinal hemorrhage is common with:
A. CRAO
B. CRVO
C. NPDR
D. papilledema

The best answer here is (b). A CRVO (central retinal vein occlusion) occurs when the primary vein draining blood from the retina becomes blocked. This results in a huge amount of blood backing up into the retina, with resulting swelling and "bruising" everywhere. This is in contrast to CRAO (central retinal artery occlusion) where blood can't even get into the eye, resulting in a pale retina. The other answers are incorrect: NPDR (non-proliferative diabetic retinopathy) occurs when diabetes causes leaky blood vessels in the retina. When severe, this can result in dot-blot hemorrhages throughout the posterior pole, but it is nowhere as impressive as with CRVO. Papilledema is swelling of the optic nerve, often from high intracranial pressure. It may cause a few hemorrhages around the nerve, but usually not extensive.

8. A "cherry red spot" in the retina is created by a:
A. lipofuscin buildup
B. histoplasmosis scar
C. choroidal hyperemia
D. axoplasmic edema

The best answer here is (d). We typically see a cherry red spot after a central retinal artery occlusion (CRAO). With this condition, the blood supply to the retina is cut off, leading to rapid damage to the retinal cells, especially the ones along the retinal surface. The superficial layer of the retina is comprised of nerve ganglion cells traveling toward the optic disc where they bundle together into the optic nerve. When these cells become hypoxic, axoplasmic flow backs up and the layer becomes white and swollen. This makes the retina look pale. The only spot that doesn't turn white is the central fovea, because there are less ganglion nerve cells here. This creates a red spot of normal colored tissue within a field of pale pink. A cherry red spot is also seen with Tay-Sachs disease. The other answers are incorrect. Histoplasmosis is contracted from chickens/bats and can create scars in the retina. Lipofuscin buildup under the retina creates the drusen that are a precursor to macular degeneration.

9. A central retinal artery occlusion might be caused by all, except:
A. arrhythmia
B. carotid blockage
C. giant cell arteritis
D. glaucoma

The best answer is (d). A CRAO has similar risks as a stroke, namely vasculopathic risk factors (high blood pressure, high cholesterol) and embolic sources (carotid plaques, heart clots). An important cause of CRAO is giant cell arteritis. This condition causes inflammation of the arteries around the head and may hit the other eye if steroids aren't used promptly. Glaucoma isn't highly associated with CRAO.

10. A patient complains of slowly decreased vision in one eye. On exam, you are unable to improve their vision despite refracting and pinholing the patient. The retina looks normal on exam, and there is no APD and confrontational fields seem normal by finger counting. The next logical step might be:
A. visual field
B. OCT
C. angiography
D. MRI

The best answer is probably (b), though (a) is also acceptable. An OCT scan of the retina is a fast, non-invasive way to check for unrecognized retinal edema. Mild retinal swelling can't always be seen during a dilated exam. A visual field test is also useful, though most neurologic changes occur suddenly or involve both eyes. More advanced investigation, such as FA (fluorescein angiography) or MRI can be considered if no other problem or localizing lesion is found.

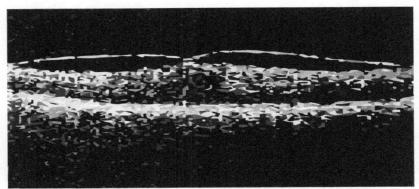

A "fast mac" OCT is performed, which shows macular traction with retinal thickening.

11. Histoplasmosis is all of the following, except:
A. contracted by inhaling spores
B. associated with chicken farmers
C. creates retinal scars
D. causes uveitis

The best answer is (d). Histoplasmosis is a fungus found in the Midwest. The fungus is found on the ground around old chicken coops and in caves harboring bats. The spores are released in the air when the ground is disturbed and then inhaled. Initial infection can cause flu-like symptoms and lung problems. In the eye, infection can cause small discreet scars in the retina. These are often described as looking "punched out." These patients can show retinal atrophy around their optic nerves and are also at higher risk for developing CNV (choroidal neovascularization), similar to wet macular degeneration. Histoplasmosis eye involvement is usually found incidentally during a routine eye exam and is thus described as POHS (presumed ocular histoplasmosis syndrome). The fungus isn't really associated with active uveitis inflammation.

12. What superhero/villain is most likely to suffer from toxoplasmosis infection?
A. Batman
B. Catwoman
C. The Penguin
D. Robin

The best answer is (b). Toxoplasmosis can be contracted from cat poop. This infection can cause internal ocular inflammation (uveitis) and is a common cause for retinal scarring.

13. What superhero/villain is most likely to suffer from histoplasmosis infection?
A. Batman
B. Catwoman
C. The Joker
D. Iron Man

The best answer here is (a). Histoplasmosis infection of the eye is common in people from the Midwest with exposure to bird poop (chickens) and bat guano. The diagnosis is described as POHS, or "presumed ocular histoplasmosis syndrome." These patients have small "punched out" scars in the retina found during an incidental eye exam.

14. Retinitis pigmentosa is a genetic disorder that:
A. affects the rods and cones
B. is autosomal dominant
C. associated with albinism
D. affects the bipolar and amacrine cells

The best answer here is (a). Retinitis pigmentosa (RP) is a genetic condition affecting the photoreceptors (usually the rods). It causes gradual and progressive vision loss, usually starting in the peripheral vision and moving centrally over many years. It is genetic and there

CHAPTER 11: RETINA

are more than 80 identified types with various inheritance patterns. RP is the leading cause for progressive blindness in young people. People with albinism also have vision problems, but this is from a lack of pigment in their retina, malformation of the macula (foveal hypoplasia) and occasionally optic nerve development issues. The intermediate cell layers (bipolar, amacrine) of the retina are not affected with RP and are of little importance to the beginning eye student.

15. Clinically significant macular edema (CSME) is classified based on the presence of any of the following, <u>except</u>:
A. macular edema
B. proximity to the fovea
C. presence of hard exudates
D. presence of neovascularization

The best answer is (d). CSME refers to swelling of the macula from diabetic vessel leakage. It is defined as having any of the following features:

1. Retinal thickening within 500 microns of the macular center

2. Hard exudates within 500 microns of the macular center with adjacent retinal thickening

3. One or more disc diameters of retinal thickening, part of which is located within one disc diameter from the macular center

CSME is an important (and testable) definition to know, especially for ophthalmology residents, though it may be a little advanced for beginning students. When a diabetic patient has CSME, it is usually treated with FLT laser or anti-VEGF medications. Neovascuariation, on the other hand, is an indicator that your patient has progressed to PDR (proliferative diabetic retinopathy). This is treated with large amounts of PRP laser applied to the peripheral retina.

16. What internal foreign substance is most toxic to the eye?
A. glass
B. plastic
C. steel
D. iron

The correct answer is (d). Iron tends to rust quickly in the saline (salt) filled interior of the eye. This is especially damaging to the retina and iron-induced inflammation is called siderosis. It typically occurs via foreign body penetration into the eye where all the fragments can't be found and removed. Plastics aren't as bad. In fact, the implants used in cataract surgery are made from acrylic plastic and are obviously well-tolerated. Glass is also inert and well tolerated. Steel isn't "good," but it breaks down slower than iron and copper.

17. All of the following may be injected into the eye in a retina doctor's office exam chair except for:
A. monoclonal antibodies
B. expanding gas bubbles
C. silicone oil
D. liquified antibiotics

The best answer is (c). Anti-VEGF medications like Avastin are actually mouse-derived monoclonal antibodies. They are commonly injected during office visits to treat wet macular degeneration. Expanding gas (SF6, C3F8) is used to treat retinal detachments via pneumatic retinopexy. This is a less aggressive treatment then taking the patient to surgery for a vitrectomy or buckle. When a patient presents with an endophthalmitis infection, antibiotics can be injected into the eye via a "tap and inject" approach. Silicone oil *can* be placed in the eye, but this is done during *surgery* and normally used for recalcitrant retinal detachments that have failed prior surgical repair.

CHAPTER 11: RETINA

18. All of the following injectable drugs were developed for treating macular degeneration, <u>except</u>:
A. Lucentis
B. Macugen
C. Eylea
D. Avastin

The best answer is (d). Avastin is an anti-VEGF medication that was originally developed and used to treat colon cancer. Tumors tend to grow fast and require a quickly growing blood supply to keep up (neovascularization). Avastin was developed to target these fast-growing vessels. The use of Avastin in the eye is considered off-label, but it is still done as this medication is inexpensive when used at the lower dosages required for the eye. The other medications are more specific anti-VEGF drugs that were made specifically for ocular use. These alternatives have less systemic side effects but are very expensive.

19. Focal laser therapy (FLT) refers to all, <u>except</u>:
A. laser near the macula
B. laser in the peripheral retina
C. laser treatment of retinal tear
D. laser treatment to decrease angiogenesis

The best answer here is (d). FLT stands for "focal laser therapy" and is a general term used to describe retina laser applied in discreet spots. This is often used to treat microaneurysms that form in diabetics with CSME. FLT can be applied to retinal tears in the periphery to keep them from progressing into full-blown detachments. This is in contrast to PRP (pan-retinal photocoagulation), which is the application of hundreds (or thousands) of laser burns to the peripheral retina. PRP is used to decrease angiogenesis (the formation of neovascular blood vessels) by sacrificing ischemic tissue to decrease VEGF hormone production. PRP is the treatment of choice for treating proliferative diabetic retinopathy. It is sometimes used to treat neovascularization from CRVO and ROP.

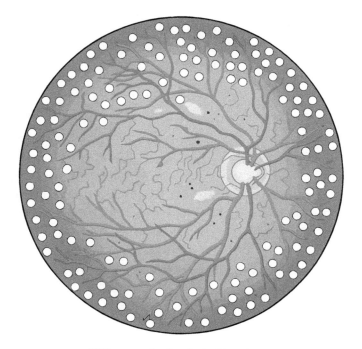

PRP laser requires hundreds of laser burns in the peripheral retina.

20. A vitrectomy might be performed for all the following, except:
A. hyphema
B. vitreous hemorrhage
C. retinal detachment
D. endophthalmitis

The best answer is (a). A vitrectomy is a retinal surgery where the vitreous gel in the back of the eye is removed. This might be done to clear out a bloody hemorrhage or debris from an active or old endophthalmitis infection. A vitrectomy is also performed during retinal detachment repair. A hyphema is a layer of blood in the anterior chamber of the eye and usually resolves without surgical intervention.

CHAPTER 11: RETINA

21. Retina laser is usually what kind of laser?
A. YAG laser
B. argon laser
C. femtosecond laser
D. excimer laser

The best answer is (b). The argon laser is used to perform FLT and PRP laser of the retina because this laser can burn and create localized scarring. The YAG laser is used on "after cataracts," and the femtosecond is used to cut LASIK flaps and create the incisions during laser cataract surgery. The excimer laser is used to ablate the corneal surface during LASIK/PRK surgery.

22. What cell type is most populous in the retina?
A. rods
B. cones
C. ganglion
D. bipolar cells

The best answer is (a). Rods are responsible for peripheral and low-light vision. They are the most populous cell type in the retina, numbering over 100 million in number. Cones, which are used for color vision and fine central acuity, number only 10 million and are concentrated around the macula. Signals from these photoreceptors are mixed down to intermediate cells such as the bipolar cells, before terminating at the ganglion cells. There are only 1.25 million ganglion cells that form the optic nerve, which illustrates that there is a certain amount of visual processing that occurs at the retinal level.

23. Fluorescein angiography (FA) is most useful for visualizing:
A. conjunctival perfusion
B. iris neovascularization
C. retinal perfusion
D. choroidal vasculature

The best answer is (c). FA is best used for visualizing retinal vasculature and perfusion. Yellow fluorescein is injected into the arm and retinal photographs are taken as the dye travels through the arteries and veins in the back of the eye. The underlying choroid can also be seen during FA, to a degree, but the choroid is better visualized with ICG (indocyanine green) angiography. There aren't many choroid eye problems, however, so ICG is rarely performed. Conjunctival perfusion is not really a problem. Iris neovascularization is an ominous sign of proliferative diabetic retinopathy (PDR) and can be seen during routine slit-lamp examination of the iris surface.

24. What power lens is typically used at the slit-lamp to visualize the retina?
A. 20 D
B. 28 D
C. 90 D
D. 98 D

The best answer is (c). The 90 diopter lens is probably the most common lens used to examine the optic nerve and posterior pole at the slit-lamp microscope. The larger 20 diopter lens is only used for indirect examination of the peripheral retina while wearing a head-mounted indirect ophthalmoscope. This is also true for the less common 28 diopter lens. To my knowledge, there is no such thing as a 98 diopter lens.

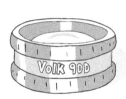
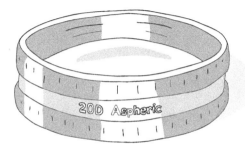

The 90 and 20 diopter lenses are the most common ones used.

CHAPTER 11: RETINA

25. Shafer's sign is only seen with:
A. rhegmatogenous retinal detachments
B. tractional retinal detachment
C. exudative retinal detachment
D. dry eye

The best answer is (a). When the retina is torn, pigment from the underlying RPE (retinal pigment epithelium) can be released to float in the vitreous cavity. This pigment can be seen floating behind the lens and is sometimes called tobacco dust or Shafer's sign. You wouldn't see this with a tractional or exudative retinal detachment as the retina is not actually torn with these entities.

26. The photoreceptors obtain their nutrition primarily from the:
A. choroid
B. central retinal vein
C. central retinal artery
D. cavernous sinus

The correct answer is (a). The blood vessels you see coursing along the surface of the retina are branches off the central retinal artery and vein that primarily feed the surface retinal cells such as the ganglion nerves. The photoreceptors, on the other hand, live deep within the retina and receive their nutrition from the choroid. The choroid is a bed of blood vessels under the retina that nourishe the overlying rods and cones and removes waste products from these cells. With a retinal detachment, the retinal photoreceptors are pulled away from the choroid bed. This causes ischemic damage to the photoreceptors within 90 minutes. This explains why the vision is so poor after "macula off" detachments are repaired.

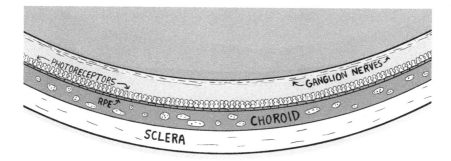

The choroid sits under the retina and provides nutrition to the deep photoreceptors.

27. Before striking the retina photoreceptors, light must pass through all of the following cell layers first, <u>except</u>:
A. ganglion nerves
B. retinal pigment epithelium
C. bipolar cells
D. amacrine cells

The correct answer is (b). The photoreceptors of the eye (rods and cones) are located at the bottom of the retina. Light must travel through a lot of other cells before striking these receptors. This includes the surface ganglion fibers and the "intermediate" retinal layers (bipolar, amacrine). The RPE layer, however, is even deeper than the photoreceptors. This layer helps transfer nutrition and waste products between the photoreceptors and the underlying choroidal vascular bed.

28. The most common type of retinal detachment is:
A. tractional
B. serous
C. effusive
D. rhegmatogenous

The correct answer is (d). A rhegmatogenous (pronounced "reg-ma-TAH-jen-us") is the classic torn retina that usually occurs after a vitreous detachment. Tractional detachments usually occur from bad proliferative diabetic retinopathy, where surface scarring and neovascular vessels tug on the retina, lifting it up. Serous detachments are rare, generally occurring from the effusion of fluid from a sub-retinal mass (tumor).

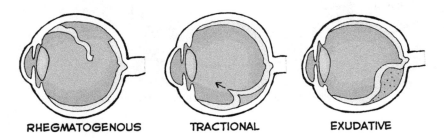

RHEGMATOGENOUS　　　TRACTIONAL　　　EXUDATIVE

29. Potential treatments for a retinal detachment <u>DON'T</u> include:
A. vitreous removal
B. silicone band
C. intraocular suture
D. gas bubble

The correct answer is (c). A retinal detachment can be repaired in several ways. The most common is a PPV (pars plana vitrectomy), where the surgeon enters the eye and removes the vitreous gel that is causing traction on the retina. The retina can then be lasered back into position. Another technique is to place a band, or "buckle" made of silicone that wraps around the outside of the eye. This band is tightened to push the scleral wall inward to reapproximate with the retina. For small superior retinal tears, a pneumatic retinopexy can be performed. This involves injecting a gas bubble into the eye that floats up and tamponades the retina into position. Intraocular sutures aren't used for retina surgery. Instead, the retina is pegged into place using laser or cryotherapy (freezing).

30. Asteroid hyalosis is:
A. a harmless cause of floaters
B. ominous
C. self-resolving
D. a popular video game

The correct answer is (a). Asteroid hyalosis are harmless calcium soap deposits that form in the vitreous. These look like white specks or snowflakes inside a snow globe. The opacities seem impressive on exam but don't cause as many visual complaints as you might expect given their dramatic appearance. Asteroid hyalosis is common, harmless, and not associated with any systemic or ocular diseases. If extremely dense, they may need to be removed with a vitrectomy (but this is rarely necessary).

31. When a retina doctor enters the eye, he or she attempts to enter through the:
A. equator
B. ora serrata
C. pars plana
D. limbus

The correct answer is (c). Retina doctors enter the eye through the pars plana. This is the flat part of the ciliary muscle, located approximately 4 mm posterior/lateral to the edge of the limbus. This entry point avoids hitting the iris and lens, while also avoiding the retina. The "equator" of the eye would be too far back to access. The ora serrata is the junction of the retina with the ciliary body (pars plana). Entrance through the ora might cause the retina to rip or disinsert at this point and cause further problems.

32. Which retinal detachment is the biggest emergency?
A. tractional
B. macula on
C. macula off

The best answer is (b). The macula is the most important part of the retina, as it is responsible for fine central vision. It is also very dependent upon the underlying choroidal bed of blood vessels for its nutrition. If the macula detaches, it loses its blood supply and permanent ischemic damage occurs within 90 minutes. There is no way to diagnose, set up surgery, and repair the retina in 90 minutes, so macula-off detachments <u>aren't</u> an emergency - the damage has already been done. These detachments are usually repaired within a week. A macula-on detachment, however, means that the detachment is still contained within the periphery. This needs to be repaired quicker, before the macula comes off as well. Tractional detachments typically occur from untreated diabetic retinopathy where neovascular scarring has slowly pulled the retina up into folds.

CHAPTER 12
TRAUMA

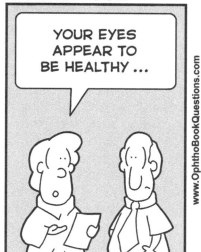
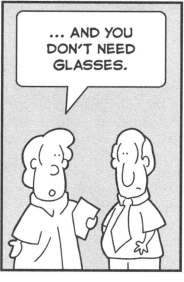
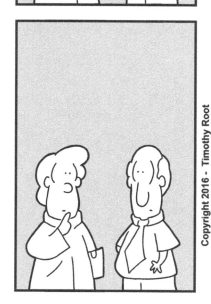
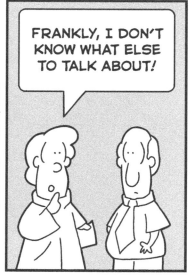

TRAUMA

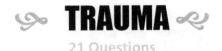

21 Questions

1. A subconjunctival hemorrhage may lead to:
A. corneal dellen
B. internal ocular bleeding
C. hyphema
D. malignancy

The best answer is (a). A subconjunctival hemorrhage occurs when one of the blood vessels in the conjunctiva skin ruptures. This can happen with trauma, with coughing, and sometimes randomly. The bleed creates an impressive amount of redness to the eye. While essentially harmless, the one complication we worry about with this is a corneal dellen. This occurs when the hemorrhage causes a raised elevation on the conjunctiva. The elevation keeps the tear film from spreading properly with blinking, creating a dry spot on the adjacent cornea. This dry spot leads to dramatic thinning of the cornea and is called a "dellen." Fortunately, these dellen respond quickly to lubrication. A subconjunctival hemorrhage is unrelated to internal eye bleeding such as hyphema. While there are a few tumors in the orbit that could cause recurrent conjunctival hemorrhage, these are extremely rare and beyond the scope of the student.

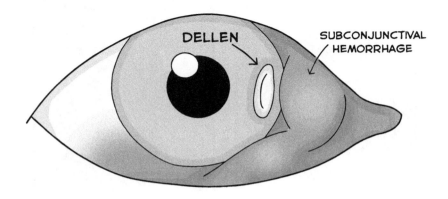

2. Removal of the contents of the eye, <u>except</u> for the sclera, is called:
A. vitrectomy
B. enucleation
C. evisceration
D. exenteration

The correct answer is (c). Generally, there are three ways to remove an eye.
1. **Enucleation** - removal of the entire eyeball
2. **Evisceration** - removing the cornea and internal eye structures (retina, iris, lens) only, leaving the scleral shell behind
3. **Exenteration** - removal of the entire orbit contents (eyeball, muscles, tissues, etc.)

A vitrectomy is removal of the vitreous jelly, usually performed during a retinal detachment repair.

3. In what condition might you remove an eye to save the other eye?
A. body dysmorphia
B. trigeminal neuralgia
C. sympathetic ophthalmia
D. Hammurabi Syndrome

The correct answer is (c). Perforating injury to an eye may release uveal tissue to the rest of the body. Our immune system is not used to this tissue and can develop an immune response to it. This causes the body to attack the uvea (choroid, iris, ciliary body) in <u>both</u> eyes. To keep this from happening, a severely traumatized eye without visual potential is removed within a few weeks of the injury. Sympathetic ophthalmia is pretty rare, however, and modern surgical technique and antibiotics have vastly improved post-traumatic visual results such that few traumatized eyes are enucleated these days. There is no such thing as Hammurabi syndrome ... Hammurabi was an ancient Babylonian king who created the first known set of laws known as the "Code of Hammurabi."

CHAPTER 12: TRAUMA

4. How frequently should patients with a hyphema be checked?
A. daily
B. weekly
C. monthly
D. yearly

The best answer is (a). Hyphema (a layer of blood in the anterior chamber) can cause high pressure in the eye. These patients need to be checked daily during the first week. After the initial bleed, a clot will form on the iris. This clot resorbs and goes away around day 3-5, leading to a rebleed and a potential spike in eye pressure. After the blood resorbs and pressure is controlled, follow-up visits can be relaxed. I will typically perform gonioscopy at one month to see if there is any trauma in the angle that might cause glaucoma problems in the future.

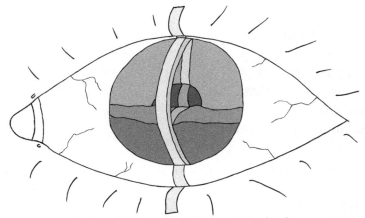

A hyphema is a layer of blood in the anterior chamber.

5. The best treatment for pressure control in a case of hyphema is:
A. anterior chamber lavage
B. timolol
C. dorzolamide
D. paracentesis

The best answer is (b). Hyphema is a layer of blood in the anterior chamber of the eye that usually occurs after trauma. Blood cells can clog the trabecular meshwork and elevate internal ocular pressure. Pressure drops like timolol may be necessary if the pressure is climbing. The carbonic anhydrase inhibitors (topical dorzolamide and oral Diamox) are normally very good agents for lowering pressure, but you have to be careful to rule out sickle cell disease first. These medications will acidify the aqueous fluid, which makes the red blood cells sickle and clog the drain even worse. Most hyphemas resolve on their own, but on rare occasions a clot can be removed with an AC washout. Very high pressure can be relieved with paracentesis. This involves using a needle or blade through the cornea to "burp" out some fluid. The AC fluid refills rapidly, however, so this really isn't a great long-term strategy. Also, the sudden pressure drop can cause a rebleed.

6. A hyphema increases the patient's long-term risk for:
A. glaucoma
B. cataracts
C. macular degeneration
D. hypopyon

The best answer is (a) though (b) is also acceptable. Any injury bad enough to cause bleeding inside the eye is likely bad enough to damage the trabecular meshwork drain and lead to glaucoma years later. The damage can be microscopic and undetectable on exam, or it may be visible as a disinsertion of the iris/ciliary muscle. In fact, a month after a hyphema injury, doctors will often perform gonioscopy to examine the angle to look for "angle recession." This is a rip within the ciliary body that looks like a dark pit and indicates a higher chance for future pressure problems. Trauma can also lead to premature cataracts, but not macular degeneration. A hypopyon is a layer of white pus inside the eye and is unrelated to hyphema.

CHAPTER 12: TRAUMA

7. An appropriate bedtime analgesic for a corneal abrasion would be:
A. tetracaine
B. proparacaine
C. loteprednol
D. artificial tears

The correct answer is (d). You <u>never</u> give a patient numbing drops (tetracaine and proparacaine) to use at home. These drops are toxic to the cornea, and will delay wound healing. The immediate pain relief will encourage the patient to use them constantly, and they'll end up with a huge corneal ulcer. Steroids, such as prednisilone and loteprednol, are also bad ideas, since they drastically increase the chance of infection when you have an open wound. For pain control, you can prescribe oral pain medicines, artificial tears, bandage contact lens, and possibly short-term patching. A cycloplegic dilating drop like homatropine can help with photophobia by paralyzing the iris muscle to keep it from "spasming."

8. A full-thickness cornea perforation can be detected using what test:
A. Schirmer's test
B. Seidel test
C. Schilling test
D. Seinfeld test

The correct answer is (b). With the Seidel test, you wipe a fluorescein strip over a suspected corneal perforation to see if aqueous fluid is oozing out through the wound. This is similar to pouring water over a bicycle/car tire to locate an air leak. The Schirmer test uses paper strips to measure dry eye. The Schilling test is used to detect problems with B12 vitamin deficiency from pernicious anemia in the stomach/intestines. There is no Seinfeld test unless you are into TV trivia.

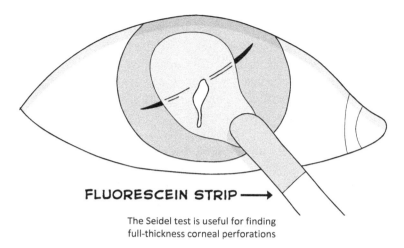

FLUORESCEIN STRIP ⟶

The Seidel test is useful for finding full-thickness corneal perforations

9. Corneal abrasions should be examined how soon after instilling fluorescein?
A. immediately
B. 1 minute
C. 2 minutes
D. 5 minutes

The best answer is (a). It is easiest to view corneal abrasions right after instilling fluorescein, though it is still easy to view abrasions minutes afterwards. The problem with waiting is that yellow color can seep into the cornea through an abrasion and make the surrounding sclera glow. This can make it harder to see early signs of infection. In reality, abrasions are pretty easy to visualize under the microscope no matter when you put the dye in.

10. The most troubling eyelid lacerations occur near the:
A. lateral canthus
B. medial canthus
C. orbital rim
D. tragus

CHAPTER 12: TRAUMA

The correct answer is (b). The medial canthus is the corner of the eyelids where they join near the nose. A lid laceration here is vexing, because the lacrimal drainage system (punctum and canaliculi) are here and may be damaged. If this system scars down, then tears can't drain into the nose properly. When repairing medial lacerations, an attempt to identify the canaliculi is made and a silicone tube is stented through it before sewing the eyelid together. This stent is yanked out a few months later and, hopefully, the canaliculus stays open. The lateral canthus has few vital structures, nor does the skin near the orbital rim. The tragus is part of the external ear that keeps your earbud headphones from popping out.

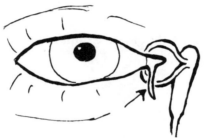

A laceration through the canaliculus can affect the tear drainage pathway.

11. What orbital wall is most likely to fracture after a blunt injury to the eye?
A. roof
B. medial wall
C. floor
D. lateral wall

The correct answer is (c). Despite the medial wall being the thinnest, it is actually the orbital floor that breaks the most often with blunt trauma. These "floor fractures" are common and rarely require repair unless the inferior rectus muscle becomes trapped or too much tissue herniates into the maxillary sinus to cause enophthalmos (a sunken-in eye).

12. What would indicate the potential need for a floor fracture repair?
A. proptosis
B. loss of cheek sensation
C. increased eye pressure
D. bradycardia

The best answer is (d). If a rectus muscle becomes entrapped in a "trap door" fracture, irritation on the muscle can induce an oculocardiac reflex and slow the heart rate. Other indicators for repair include muscle entrapment and enophthalmus (sunken-in eye). The V2 nerve runs along the orbital floor, such that many people with a floor fracture lose sensation along their cheek under the eye. This isn't an indicator for repair as most floor fractures heal spontaneously.

13. With an orbital wall fracture, how is muscle entrapment best detected?
A. forced ductions
B. motility assessment
C. presence of diplopia
D. loss of extreme gaze

The best answer is (a). With a floor fracture, a muscle can become trapped in the break and lead to motility issues. As an eye doctor, you will be asked to detect entrapment of the rectus muscles because this might require surgery with an oculoplastics or ENT doctor. Entrapment is detected with "forced ductions" which involves numbing the eye, grabbing the eye with forceps near the limbus, and manually moving the globe in all directions. A tethered muscle will keep the eye from rotating in the opposite direction. While this test sounds good in theory, it is very hard to perform on an awake patient and is something best left for the operating room or under sedation. Many patients with a wall fracture will have double vision and limited eye mobility on extreme gaze, without actually having entrapment. This motility problem occurs from temporary swelling of the eye muscles and periorbital tissue. The doubling typically goes away after a few weeks; if it doesn't, you may need to reassess and re-image to rule out muscle entrapment.

14. Potential treatments for a retrobulbar hemorrhage is:
A. lateral canthotomy
B. medial canthotomy
C. lateral wall decompression
D. retrobulbar block

The best answer is (a). A retrobulbar hemorrhage is bleeding behind the eye into the retrobulbar space. The eye socket doesn't have room to expand, so bleeding forces the eye to protrude forward. If eyelid swelling keeps the eye and orbital contents from expanding forward, a localized compartment syndrome develops and pressure buildup causes glaucomatous nerve damage. In these cases, a lateral canthotomy is performed. This involves cutting the lower lateral eyelid insertion from the bone, releasing the eyelid to allow the eye to proptose forward. You wouldn't perform this on the medial canthus, as this would be hard to access and would damage the canaliculi tear-drainage pathway. On rare occasions, oculoplastics doctors could create a floor fracture to allow more expansion into the maxillary sinus, but this would NOT be done laterally through the tough zygomatic bone. A retrobulbar block might actually CAUSE a retrobulbar hemorrhage. When we perform a block prior to cataract surgery, we apply pressure to the eye for several minutes using a Honan balloon to decrease the chance of this bleeding.

15. Treatment for a traumatic iritis may include all of the following, except:
A. topical steroid
B. dilating drops
C. oral steroids
D. glaucoma drops

The best answer is (c). Traumatic iritis typically occurs after blunt trauma to the eye and causes pain and sensitivity to light (photophobia). We generally treat this with topical steroids and cycloplegic dilating drops for pain. Dilating drops also decrease the chance of iris synechae (scar) formation along the pupil edge. Oral steroids aren't particularly helpful for intraocular inflammation. Glaucoma drops may be necessary if the pressure elevates (secondary to inflammatory blockage of the trabecular meshwork), though usually the pressure is low secondary to inflammation of the ciliary body (which produces aqueous fluid).

16. Ominous signs after a chemical burn include all, <u>except</u>:
A. cloudy cornea
B. particulate debris
C. blanched conjunctiva
D. hyperemic conjunctiva

The best answer is (d). Chemical burns to the eye can have serious consequences. With severe burns, the cornea will be cloudy and the conjunctiva white, as the conjunctival blood vessels have been burned or "cooked" off. Oddly enough, a red eye is actually a good sign following chemical injury, as this indicates that the conjunctival vessels are present. During your exam, check the pH of the eye with filter paper and make sure there isn't any debris in the eye from which more acid/base may be seeping from.

17. Initial open globe management includes the following, <u>except</u>:
A. eye pressure check
B. vision assessment
C. CT scan
D. oral antibiotics

The best answer is (a). When you have a known open globe, you don't want to push on the eye to check the pressure. This kind of palpation can expulse the contents of the eye. You do, however, want to document the vision if possible, as this is prognostic of their final outcome and may determine whether you attempt a repair or (rarely) perform enucleation. CT scans can help determine if there are any foreign bodies in the eye. They are also helpful for detecting an open globe in cases where the perforation can't be seen, such as expulsion under the rectus muscle insertions. Oral antibiotics and tetanus shots are always a good idea in these cases.

18. The initial treatment for a chemical injury to the eye is:
A. irrigation
B. vision assessment
C. sterile sand
D. buffered solution

The best answer is (a). When you get chemicals in the eye, the priority is to wash them out as quickly as possible. This takes priority over everything else, including examination. If a patient calls from home, instruct them to flush the eyes with saline or water immediately. If in the emergency room, they should do the same thing and may even use a Morgan lens for this purpose. A Morgan lens looks like a clear shell that IV tubing can be connected to it. The eye is numbed up with tetracaine and the shell is placed in the eye like an oversized contact lens. Several liters of saline are run through the lens to bath the eye and wash away chemical residue. There is no such thing as sterile sand or buffered solution for the eye.

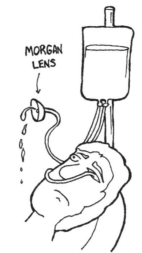

The Morgan lens is used by ER doctors in the emergency room.

19. Ruptures to the eye tend to occur at:
A. limbus
B. optic nerve insertion
C. equator
D. cornea

The best answer is (a). Blunt force trauma tends to rupture the eyeball at two places: the limbus (the cornea/sclera junction) and underneath the rectus muscle insertions. The white sclera is about 1 mm thick, except at the muscle insertions, where it is only one-third of that thickness. A rupture here is particularly challenging, as you usually can't see it directly and may have to cut back the conjunctival tissue to "explore" for it. Ruptures at the equator are unlikely and would be challenging to repair. The optic nerve can disinsert from the back of the eye; this is called an optic nerve avulsion and is rare. The cornea is pretty tough and rarely splits from blunt force alone.

CHAPTER 12: TRAUMA

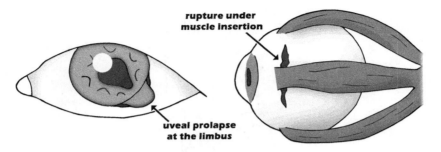

With blunt trauma, the eye tends to perforate at the limbus and under the muscle insertion points.

20. Prosthetic eyes have a shape that is:
A. spherical like a ball
B. a hemisphere
C. curved like a shell
D. thin like a contact

The best answer is (c). Unlike movie props, a prosthetic eye is usually shaped like a thick shell (not round like a marble). When we remove an eye (enucleation), we replace the eye with a spherical piece of plastic and sew the rectus muscles around it, covering the whole mess with conjunctival skin. A conformer, which looks like a clear shell, is placed on top of the conjunctiva as the tissue heals. This plastic spacer keeps the skin on the back of the eyelids from scarring down and maintains a "pocket." A custom prosthetic shell can be placed in this pocket later on.

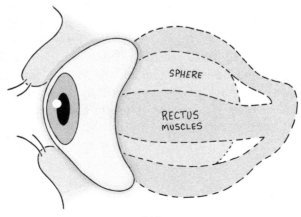

21. The best method to rule out intraocular metal foreign body is:
A. CT
B. MRI
C. x-ray
D. ultrasound

The best answer is (a). The best way to detect a small metal foreign body is with thin-slice CT of the orbit. MRI is contraindicated as the spinning magnets might turn a piece of metal into a projectile. X-ray used to be the preferred method, but it is difficult to localize metal on x-ray (skull x-rays aren't done that often these days).

CHAPTER 13
UVEITIS

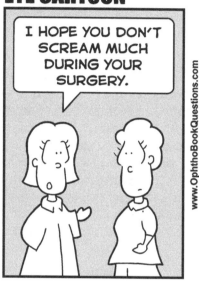
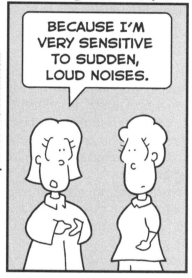
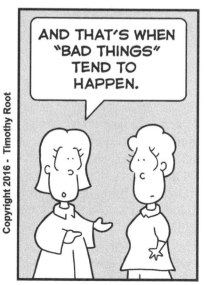

UVEITIS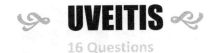

16 Questions

1. Signs of internal inflammation include:
A. photophobia
B. exophthalmos
C. enophthalmos
D. photopsia

The best answer is (a). Photophobia is sensitivity to light and is common with inflammation inside the eye. The iris muscle, which constricts based on ambient lighting, becomes sore and can "spasm" when looking at bright lights. This causes eye pain. We often treat photophobia with dilating drops to paralyze the iris muscle. This effectively immobilizes the muscle, much like putting a cast on a broken arm to immobilize it. "Exophthalmos" is when the eye protrudes forward. The term is used specifically to describe proptosis from thyroid disorder. Enophthalmos is a sinking in of the eye, such as after a floor fracture. Photopsia is seeing sparkling lights.

2. Which inflammation is deepest?
A. scleritis
B. episcleritis
C. conjunctivitis

The best answer is (a). Scleritis is a deep inflammation of the white sclera that makes up the wall of the eye. This is rare, but causes an aching pain, and is often accompanied by signs of inflammation inside the eye such as cell and flare. Scleritis is associated with pro-inflammatory conditions like rheumatoid arthritis and can be dangerous if the sclera perforates. Conjunctivitis, sometimes called "pink eye," is an inflammation of the conjunctival tissue that lies on top of the eye. The episclera is the intermediate layer of tissue and blood vessels on top of the sclera (but still under the conjunctival surface). Episcleritis tends to cause a focal area of hyperemia with dilation of deep vessels.

3. Episcleritis can be differentiated from conjunctivitis using:
A. fluorescein
B. phenylephrine
C. atropine
D. lissamine green

The best answer is (b). Episcleritis is deeper than surface conjunctivitis and involves dilation of deep blood vessels on the eye. Phenylephrine is a stimulant eye drop that we use when dilating the eye. It also tends to constrict blood vessels on the conjunctiva. If this topical phenylephrine fails to blanch a pink eye, then you may be dealing with a deeper episcleritis. Another hint is to push on the eye/eyelid with a cotton swab to see if the blood vessels move (conjunctiva is relatively loose and will move, while episcleral vessels are adherent to the sclera underneath and stay stationary). Of the other choices: fluorescein is used to check pressure and detect abrasions, atropine is a long-acting cycloplegic dilator, and lissamine green sticks to irritated cells and is used by cornea doctors looking for dry eye.

4. Limbal injection is often a sign of:
A. viral conjunctivitis
B. bacterial conjunctivitis
C. viral keratitis
D. anterior uveitis

The best answer is (d). Interior eye inflammation, such as uveitis/iritis, tends to inflame the blood vessels in a ring bordering the limbus (where the cornea inserts on the sclera). The other choices tend to inflame the entire conjunctiva.

5. Keratic precipitates are indicators of:
A. asteroid hyalosis
B. vitreous detachment
C. anterior chamber inflammation
D. chemosis

CHAPTER 13: UVEITIS

The best answer is (c). KP (keratic precipitates) are spots of debris found on the inside of the cornea that occur from inflammation inside the eye. We see this with inflammation such as uveitis/iritis, and occasionally after trauma or surgery. Asteroid hyalosis is harmless calcium soap deposits that form in the vitreous causing floaters. A vitreous detachment causes flashes and floaters, while chemosis is swelling of the conjunctiva and very common with allergic conjunctivitis.

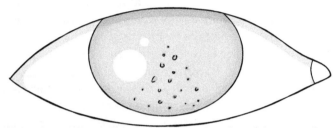

KP look like specks of mud splattered againt the inside surface of the cornea. Convection currents inside the anterior chamber will often cause the KP to form in a triangular pattern called "Arlt's triangle."

6. What <u>isn't</u> part of the uvea?
A. retina
B. iris
C. choroid
D. ciliary body

The best answer is (a). The uvea is composed of the iris, ciliary body, and the choroid. These three structures are embryologically related and are susceptible to inflammation. Uveitis is the term used to describe inflammation of these structures, although it is rare to have all three structures inflamed at the same time. More commonly, patients present with either an anterior uveitis of the iris and ciliary body, or a rare posterior uveitis of the choroid. There are many systemic causes of uveitis, including inflammatory syndromes (sarcoidosis, rheumatoid arthritis, ankylosing spondylitis) and infections (toxoplasmosis, syphilus, Lyme, TB). Most cases are idiopathic with no underlying cause identified. The term "iritis" is another way to describe anterior uveitis, though iritis is more often used in the context of "traumatic iritis."

OPHTHOBOOK QUESTIONS - VOL 1

7. Dilating drops are used with iritis to:
A. decrease pain
B. immobilize the iris
C. break synechiae
D. all of the above

The correct answer is (d). Dilating drops are useful in cases of uveitis/iritis. They help with pain by paralyzing the iris and ciliary body muscles to keep them from "spasming" with light exposure. The dilation can help avoid synechiae (scar) formation between the pupil edge and lens underneath.

8. Steroids are appropriate for treating ocular inflammation in all diseases, except:
A. sarcoidosis
B. rheumatoid arthritis
C. ankylosing spondylitis
D. toxoplasmosis

The correct answer is (d). Topical steroids are the mainstay treatment for ocular inflammation. You wouldn't use them in cases of suspected infection, however, as steroids might make an infection worse.

9. Intraocular "flare" is caused by:
A. cellular debris
B. macrophages
C. immune precipitates
D. protein

The best answer is (d). Flare looks like smoke in the anterior chamber of the eye. It is caused by protein leaking from irritated blood vessels, presumably from the iris. There isn't much significance to the presence of flare other than as a marker of inflammation. We are usually more interested in the amount of "cell" floating in the aqueous. These are cells (macrophages) and cellular debris floating in the fluid that are commonly seen after trauma, surgery, infection, and with internal ocular inflammation.

10. Appropriate uveitis lab workup includes all of the following, except:
A. RF
B. ACE
C. RPR
D. ESR

The best answer is (d). ESR is an inflammatory blood marker we obtain to rule out giant cell (temporal) arteritis. ESR isn't related to eye inflammation. The other answers are correct. Unfortunately, the blood tests we order for uveitis are pretty extensive and will require some memorization. Here are the main ones I tend to order:

SERUM LABWORK
ACE, Lysosyme (sarcoidosis)
RF (rheumatoid arthritis)
ANA (lupus)
HLA-B27 (ankylosing spondylitis, Chron's, ulcerative colitis, Reiter's, psoriatic arthritis)
Lyme titer (Lyme disease)
RPR, MHA-ATP, FTA-Abs (syphilus)
Toxoplasmosis IgG, IgM

OTHER POTENTIAL TESTS:
PPD (tuberculosis)
CXR (sarcoidosis)
X-Ray of spine and pelvis (ankylosing spondylitis)

11. Uveitis can cause pressure spikes via all, <u>except</u>:
A. inflammation of ciliary body
B. iris synechiae
C. clogged trabecular mesh work
D. iris bombe

The best answer is (a). Inflammation of the ciliary body usually decreases aqueous production and <u>lowers</u> pressure. If the pressure is elevated, it is often from TM (trabecular meshwork) irritation (a trabeculitis) or TM "clogging" from inflammatory debris. Internal eye inflammation tends to make the iris muscle "sticky" with a tendency to scar down to nearby structures. This can occur at the pupil margin and is called posterior iris synechae. If the synechae sticks the entire pupil margin down, then this will cause pressure to build up in the posterior chamber and create iris bombe (acute glaucoma attack).

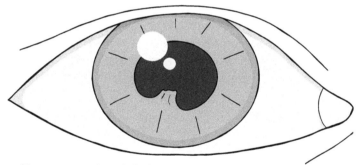

Iris synechia can create an irregularly shaped pupil. If this synechia occurs around the entire pupil margin, iris bombe occurs as aqueous can't flow forward into the anterior chamber.

12. Traumatic iritis and microhyphema can sometimes be differentiated using:
A. bright white light
B. neutral density filter
C. cobalt blue filter
D. red-free filter

CHAPTER 13: UVEITIS

The best answer is (d). The red-free filter turns the white light of the slit-lamp microscope green. Red blood cells floating in the aqueous fluid are pretty easy to see, but they disappear when you shoot green light as them because there is no red light to bounce off of them to detect (I hope that makes sense). White blood cells and macrophages (such as after a traumatic iritis) are still visible with the red-free (green) filter. In reality, <u>all</u> cells are extremely hard to see under the microscope and this red-free filter technique is not as useful as you might think.

13. The most common cause of uveitis is:
A. lupus
B. tuberculosis
C. HLA-B27 arthritis
D. syphilis

The best answer is (c). Of the choices offered, the HLA-B27 arthritis, especially ankylosing spondylitis, is the most common cause of uveitis. While lupus is common, uveitis is rare from this condition. Tuberculosis and syphilis are quite rare to begin with. Overall, most cases of uveitis are idiopathic with no underlying disease process.

14. Physical signs of an anterior uveitis include all of the following <u>except</u>:
A. ciliary injection
B. pupil dilation
C. pupil constriction
D. synechiae

The best answer is (b). Uveitis is internal inflammation inside the eye. This tends to cause ciliary injection. This can be seen as a flush of redness on the conjunctiva around the limbus. You also tend to see pupil constriction and synechiae (adhesions) between the inflamed iris and the lens underneath. It is rare to find pupil dilation as part of uveitis. In fact, we <u>like</u> to dilate these eyes, in order to avoid synechae formation and to help with pain.

15. Indications for eye removal of a phthisical eye include everything, except:
A. sympathetic ophthalmia
B. pain
C. cosmesis
D. tumor

The best answer is probably (a). A phthisical eye is an essentially blind eye that has stopped working and begun to scar down from disuse. The blindness can be from chronic retinal detachment, end-stage glaucoma, prior trauma, or congenital malformation. It takes several years for phthisis to occur, but typically the cornea will cloud over, conjunctival vessels will grow over the cornea, and the anterior chamber will flatten. Calcium deposits can form on the corneal surface. This is called "band keratopathy" and can be painful if it causes recurrent abrasions. These eyes can be painful if the pressure builds up inside. A blind, painful eye does the patient no good and is reasonable for removal. Cosmetically, a ptysical eye can be removed for better fitting of a prosthetic. Sympathetic ophthalmia is a bilateral inflammation of the uveal tissue that occurs after penetrating trauma to an eye. To avoid this, severely traumatized eyes are sometimes enucleated within 14 days of the insult to protect the good eye. This isn't relevant here, as it requires several years for phthisis to form and late removal wouldn't have any benefit in regards to sympathetic ophthalmia.

16. A layer of pus inside the eye is called:
A. hyphema
B. hypopyon
C. hyperion
D. hippopion

The correct answer is (b). A layer of inflammation or "pus" in the anterior chamber is called a hypopyon. They can occur from internal endophthalmitis infection, or as a sterile "reactive" inflammation from a surface corneal ulcer. Bad cases of uveitis can cause a

CHAPTER 13: UVEITIS

hypopyon as well. A hyphema is a layer of blood in the anterior chamber. Hyperion is a figure from ancient Greek mythology. There is no such thing of hippopion. If there was, it would be a layer of hippos.

CONCLUSION

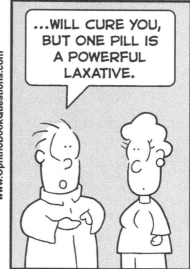
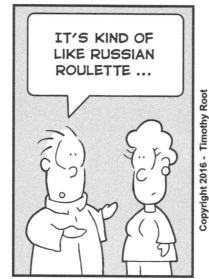
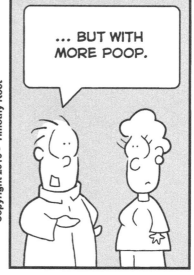

CONCLUSION

Thank you for reading this book. Hopefully, you found these questions interesting and the difficulty at an appropriate level.

The eye is a fascinating organ to study, especially when the basics are presented correctly. I attempted to keep this material high-yield for you without too much minutia.

I'd also like to thank those of you who bought the printed version of this book. Royalties from these sales allow me to keep the website up and functioning.

If you have comments about any of these questions, drop by our website (OphthoBook.com) and leave a message on the appropriate page! Also, feel free to share the free PDF version of this book with your friends and colleagues!

You can get involved with Volume 2!

This book took me a long time to write, as most of my time is spent advancing my private practice and raising my children. It may take me a few years to finish Volume 2. However, if you are interested in participating in this project, I am always looking for co-authors.

This is a great way to advance the ocular education of your peers (and to earn a chapter publication for your resume, if you need that kind of thing). Contact me at OphthoBook if you are a medical student or resident and if this is something you are interested in working on together!

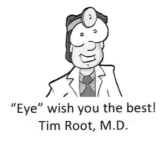

"Eye" wish you the best!
Tim Root, M.D.

CPSIA information can be obtained
at www.ICGtesting.com
Printed in the USA
LVHW092203060120
642737LV00001B/201/P